praise for
strala yoga

"Radiant well-being is a practice, not a destination.
And there's no better guide than my dear friend Tara Stiles.
In her new book *Strala Yoga*, she shares a gentle process of meditation in motion
to help turn on our relaxation response and ignite our most awakened selves.
Get your Strala on to simmer in the good, healing, and soulful work."

KRIS CARR
New York Times best-selling author

❁

"Tuning into intuition and gaining awareness through the moving meditation,
along with approaching challenges with ease, are a dash of the
magic ingredients that make up the special sauce of Strala Yoga.
You get more with less effort. Everyone wants that."

GABRIELLE BERNSTEIN
New York Times best-selling author of *Miracles Now*

❁

"Our sense of connection to our true inner self comes
naturally with the easygoing process of Strala Yoga. This is the yoga revolution
that readily brings spiritual practice into our everyday lives."

DR. RUDY TANZI
New York Times best-selling author of *Super Brain* and *Super Genes*

❁

"Practicing Strala's principles of ease and natural movement helps us
not only become strong and balanced in our body and mind, but also maintain
a deep connection to accomplishing challenges with ease in our lives."

JASON WACHOB
founder & CEO, mindbodygreen and author of *Wellth*

❁

"Strala Yoga is a wonderful practice to release physical and
emotional tension and come back to our energized, balanced, happy state.
I love attending Strala classes to move freely, gain physical capability,
and enjoy the process of moving how it feels good in my body."

JESSICA ORTNER
New York Times best-selling author of
The Tapping Solution for Weight Loss and *Body Confidence*

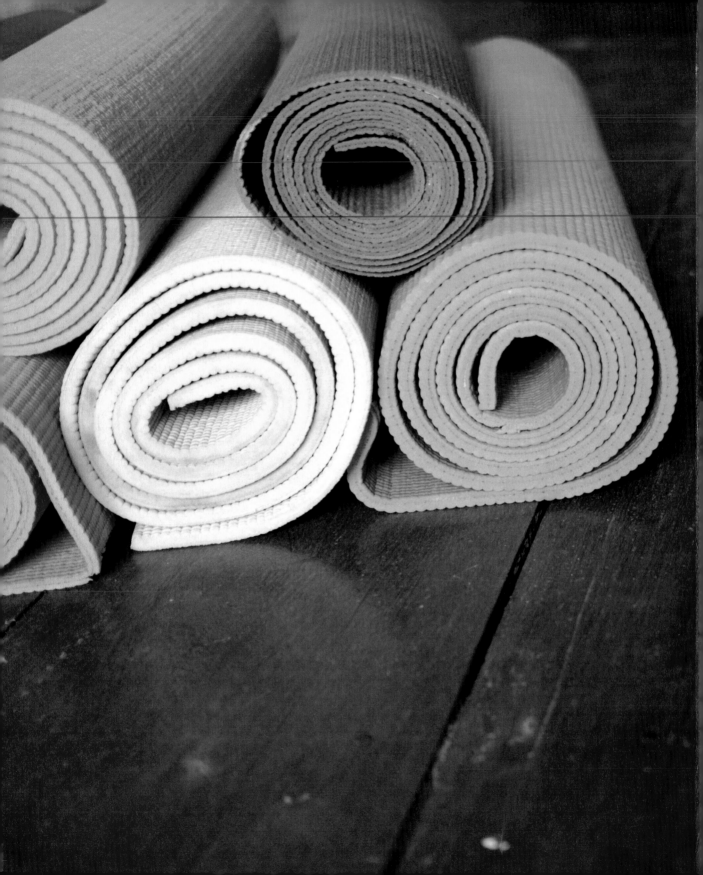

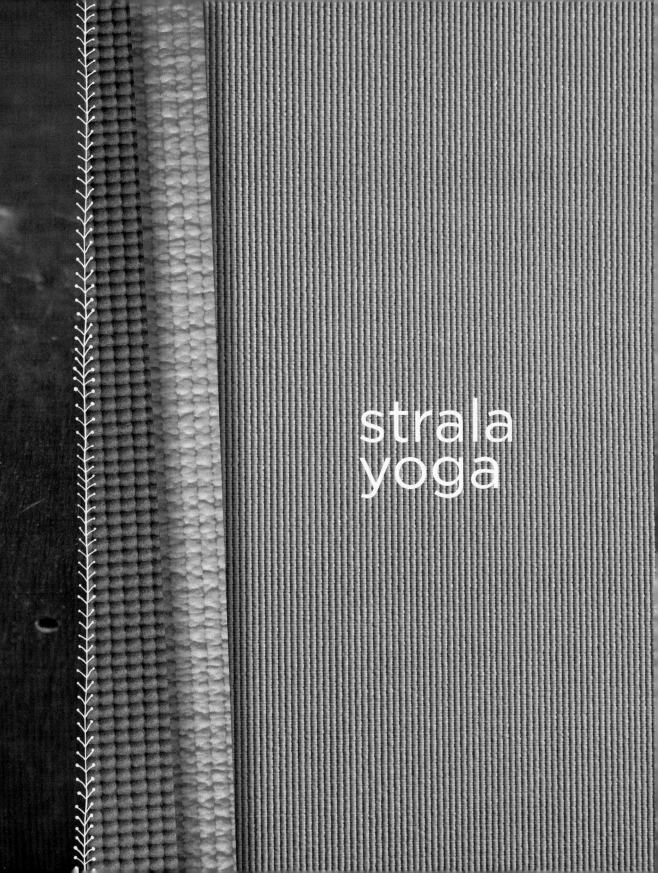

strala
yoga

ALSO BY TARA STILES

MAKE YOUR OWN RULES COOKBOOK:
More Than 100 Simple, Healthy Recipes
Inspired by Family and Friends Around the World

MAKE YOUR OWN RULES DIET

SLIM CALM SEXY YOGA:
210 Proven Yoga Moves for Mind/Body Bliss

YOGA CURES:
Simple Routines to Conquer
More Than 50 Ailments and Live Pain-Free

TARA STILES

best-selling author of *Yoga Cures*

strala yoga

Be Strong, Focused
& Ridiculously Happy
from the Inside Out

 HAY HOUSE, INC.

Carlsbad, California ☆ New York City
London ☆ Sydney ☆ Johannesburg
Vancouver ☆ New Delhi

Published and distributed in the United States by: Hay House, Inc.: www.hayhouse.com®
Published and distributed in Australia by: Hay House Australia Pty. Ltd.: www.hayhouse.com.au
Published and distributed in the United Kingdom by: Hay House UK, Ltd.: www.hayhouse.co.uk
Published and distributed in the Republic of South Africa by: Hay House SA (Pty.), Ltd.: www.hayhouse.co.za
Distributed in Canada by: Raincoast Books: www.raincoast.com
Published in India by: Hay House Publishers India: www.hayhouse.co.in

book design
Charles McStravick

Photo Credits
Photos on pages ii, iii, iv, vi, viii, ix, x, 1, 4, 5, 6, 7, 8, 9, 13, 14, 15, 28, 31, 32,
33, 36, 38, 68, 72, 100, 108, 140, 146, 148, 149, 150, 161, 169, 194, 202, 203,
218, 225, 232, 264, 266, 267, 268, 269, 280, 316, 318, 320, 322, 323, 324, 325,
326, and 328 by under license from Shutterstock.com

Yoga routine photos courtesy of Thomas Hoeffgen.

All other photos courtesy of Tara Stiles

Cataloging-in-Publication Data is on file at the Library of Congress

Tradepaper ISBN: 978-1-4019-4812-2

10 9 8 7 6 5 4 3 2 1
1st edition, August 2016

PRINTED IN THE UNITED STATES OF AMERICA

FOR CHRISTINE ZILKA & PENNY,
WHO REMIND US THAT
EASE OF BODY AND MIND
DOES WONDERS FOR
PRETTY MUCH EVERYTHING.

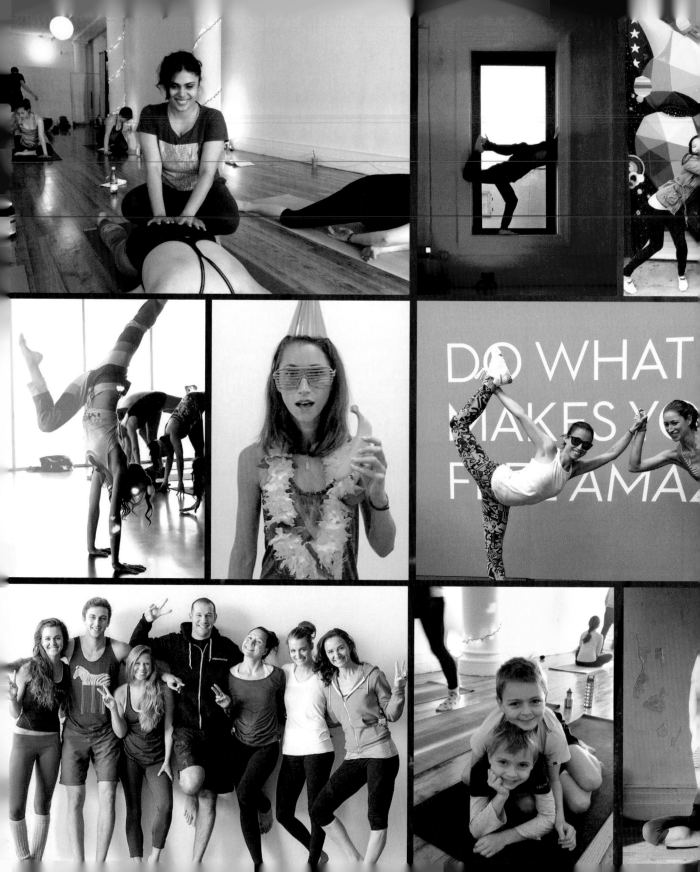

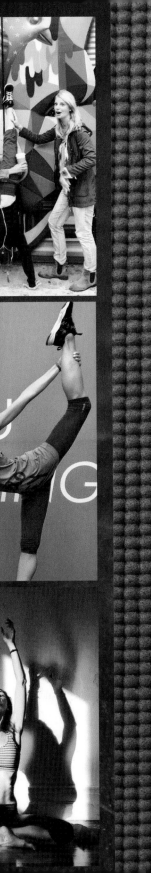

contents

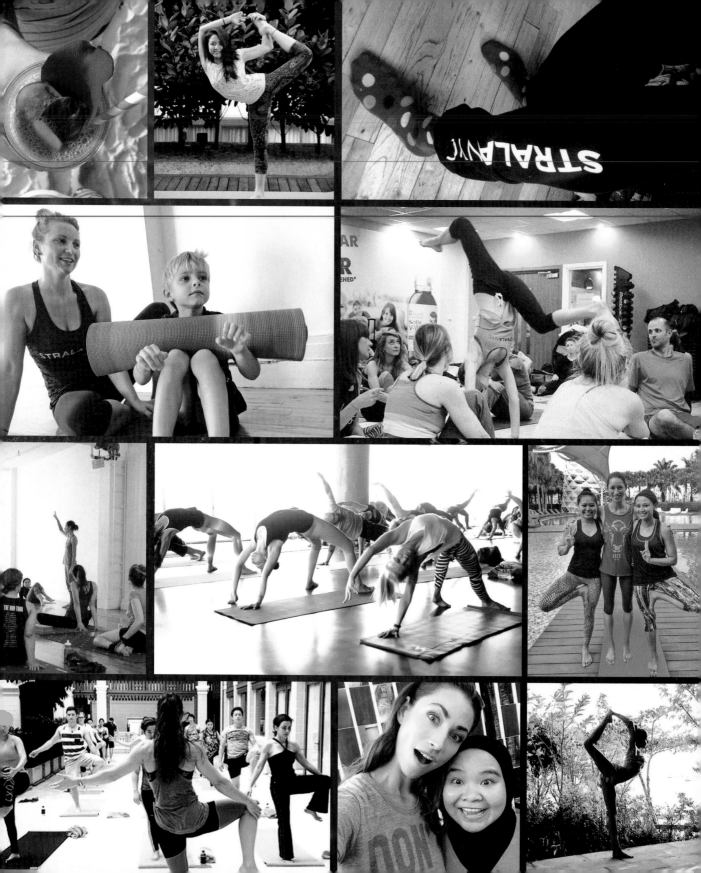

INTRODUCTION

Do you want to feel fantastic? Of course you do!

We all do. Luckily, there is a way to live each moment of your life feeling strong, energized, inspired, calm, focused, and ridiculously happy from the inside out. And that's what I'm here to talk about.

What I've found, through my own personal exploration, is that tension is the basis of a life that feels out of whack. It's what makes you tired and irritable. Sad and stuck. Frustrated and angry. It's even what makes you get that mediocre meh feeling. Life doesn't have to be terrible to be not fantastic.

For years, my life was fine . . . but not amazing. I spent ages digging around, trying to find my purpose, achieve something, and find meaning. And during this time, I realized that I was carrying around bucket loads of tension. I thought I was chill, easygoing, an attractor for all the things I desired, but I seemed to never get what I wanted. Why wasn't everything showing up for me? I worked hard. I followed the rules. But my efforts weren't adding up to results. What was I doing wrong?

After attempting to work through what was holding me back, something gradually—and then suddenly—shifted in my body. I realized that I needed to use my energy in a more effective way. I didn't know how to do that, but I knew I needed to change. I felt an inexplicable sense of urgency to take myself off my current path and find a better way. I just wasn't sure how.

After years of play and exploration, I discovered that the better way was a path of ease. Not the easiest path, but a path where we approach any situation from a place of calm, wise ease. With ease, we can let go of the tension that squashes our intuition, physical and mental ability, and creativity. We are able to let go of the blocks that keep us stranded in one place. We experience freedom and space.

The discovery of ease was a long process, but it led to the creation of Strala Yoga—which is something I will be eternally grateful for. Strala is a philosophy of movement that takes you back to yourself. It isn't about strict rules or sets of poses. It's about feeling and intuition and natural movement. It's all about the "how" of moving instead of the "what." The classes of Strala focus on moving how it feels good for you instead of on moving into certain poses. They are about lingering where it feels good to linger and breathing your way through difficult moments instead of forcing yourself into rigid poses. Strala classes are about the freedom to move in your own way—without the pressure of rules.

Since I started teaching this form of yoga, I've seen thousands of people take the freedom and ease they've been practicing in class with them into their lives. They feel healthier and happier. They ditch the stress and are able to laugh off things that used to drive them crazy. They have easier and more fun interactions with their colleagues and friends. They search out and enjoy healthier foods and activities. All in all, life just gets better. When you practice ease regularly on the mat, it becomes a habit off the mat. And that's when life gets really good. This book is about how to do just that.

My goal is to guide you through the philosophy and movements in Strala Yoga very clearly and then simply get out of the way so you can experience how awesome and capable you are. I'm not here to be a guru. My midwestern family would smack me upside my head if I started acting more evolved or better than anyone, and frankly I know better. I'm simply here to show you how this supersustainable practice of feeling fantastic can easily fit into your life. We're headed together on a journey of fun, exploration, and ease of body and mind.

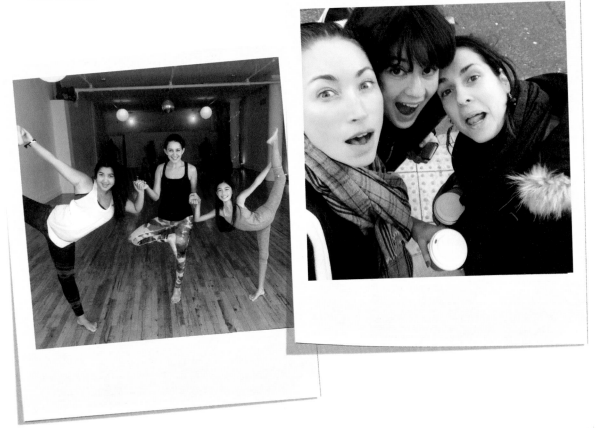

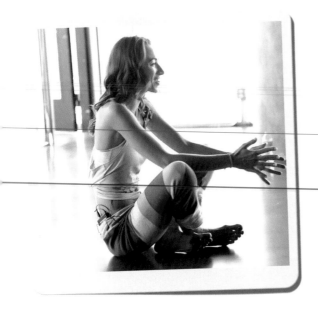

In the first part of this book, we cover the creation of Strala and dive more into the effects of tension and ease. Then we walk through the basic principles that help you create ease in your life: the breath-body connection, the importance of feeling, and the use of natural movement. After setting up a home practice using the advice in Chapter 5, you can try out 1 (or all!) of the 10 routines found in Part Two. There are photos throughout to help you along the way. (You'll notice that the angle of my pose varies in some routines—don't feel like you need to move your body 360 degrees to complete the pose! The important thing is to notice the general body position and placement of your feet and hands.) Some are basic flow movements, while others focus on specific outcomes, such as waking up, detoxing, and getting better sleep. I've also provided two programs that can help you bring yoga into your life—a short 7-day jump start and a more comprehensive 30-day guide.

Feel free to grab a notebook and write your own thoughts as you work through the following pages. I'll be presenting you with concepts and exercises that will help you understand the philosophy and mental aspects of this practice, as well as concrete advice for putting these ideas into action. When we try on new ideas and take the time to marinate on how we feel and how we can best soak up the concepts to be useful in our own lives, magic has space to rush right in.

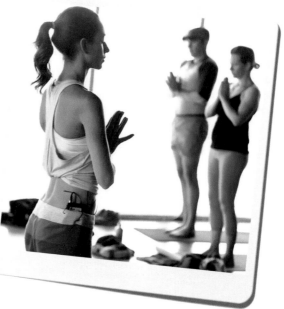

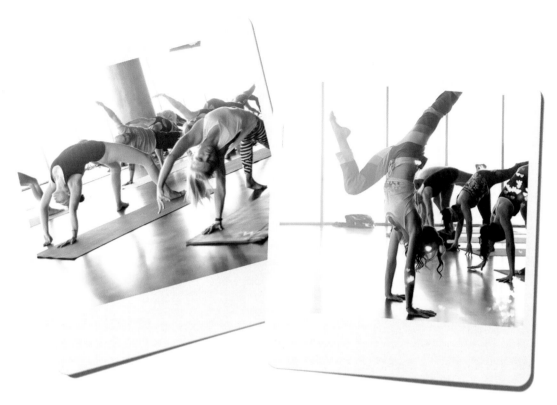

Fair warning: there is effort and focus that goes into this work, but what we can eliminate is the experience of tension, struggle, and, most important, fear. You have to show up for yourself. And you have to keep showing up. You have to practice, but you will enjoy the process. This isn't about no pain, no gain. It's about accomplishing a lot with as little effort as possible to leave loads of room for possibilities, healing, intuition, and clarity. With this process and the practice of ease, you'll realign with what's natural, work toward balancing your imbalanced areas, get more done with less effort, and have a whole lot of fun in the process.

This all sounds like a huge, ridiculous promise, right? Yeah, I know it's a lot, but I've seen countless successes—everything from the healing of physical and emotional maladies to big life transformations, including my own. The promise is in the process and commitment to yourself. If you commit to regularly practicing with ease, you will gain strength and radiant health, and you will feel fantastic, calm, clear, and connected. Basically, you will feel like the very best version of you. So get ready to feel amazing, and enjoy the ride!

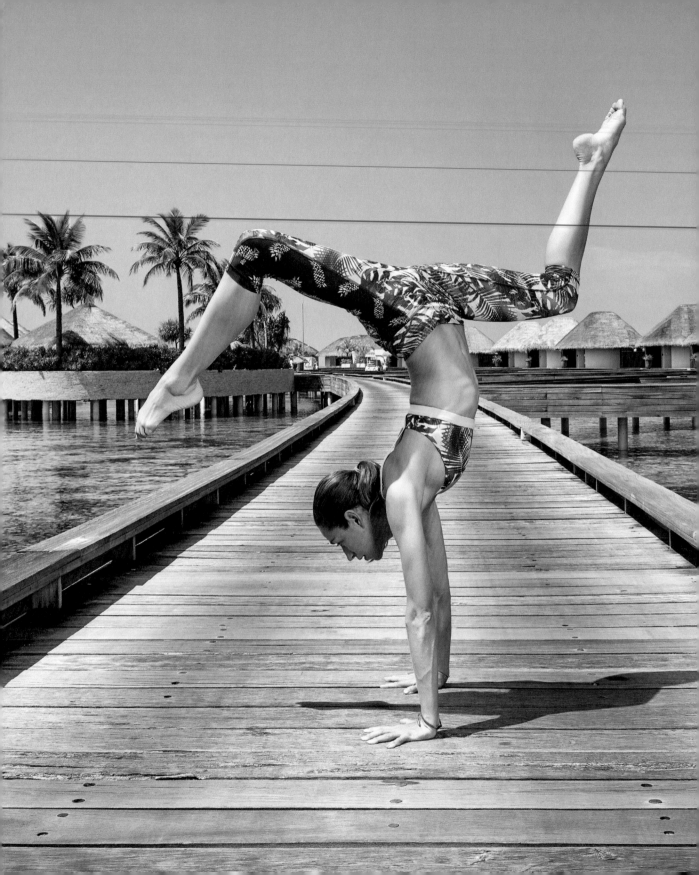

PART
ONE

move
with ease

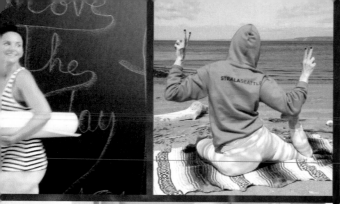
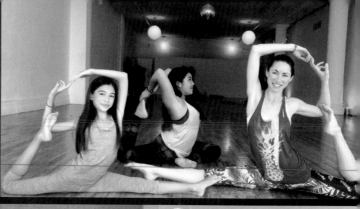
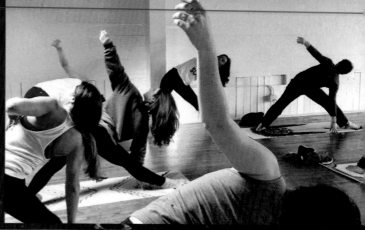
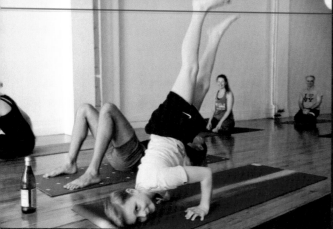
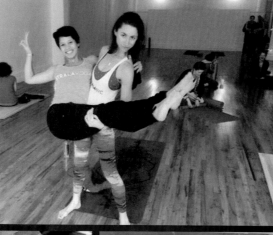
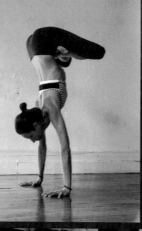
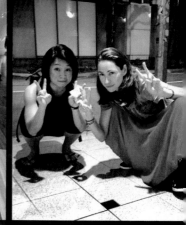
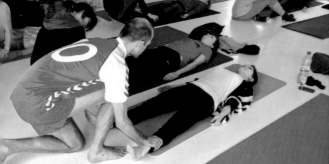
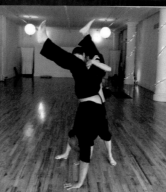
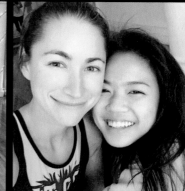

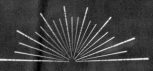

CHAPTER 1

DISCOVER EASE

the strala philosophy

The first time I saw Yoga Man I was 18 years old and part of a troupe of contemporary dancers studying at the Barat Conservatory. Our ballet teacher, Rory Foster of American Ballet Theatre, had convinced the lot of us to attend a yoga class by promising relaxation and the "prevention and repair of soreness"—promises that sounded great to me. I always hurt. My hamstrings were tight. My legs ached. I was sore and tense, so if this could help me feel better, I was totally in.

When I walked into my first yoga class, I spotted Yoga Man sitting cross-legged on the floor in the front of the room. He was tall with big, curly hair that stood out proud as an extension of his spine. His body was open and strong. He had a smile from ear to ear, and his knees were casually resting on the floor. Everything about him said, "All is well." He was patiently waiting, unaffected by the noise and the chatter, for the gaggle of us giggly dancers to roll in. It was clear from how we ignored him that none of us really cared about yoga. Most of us were only there to impress our teacher. But through the chaos and even arrogance that accompanied our arrival, he just sat, so darn naturally happy.

I was overwhelmed by his presence. All I could think was, *How can this guy not be stressed? How can his life be so great that he's happy teaching yoga to a bunch of distracted dancers?* I was stressed out *for* him. Later I came to realize that Yoga Man embodied what was missing in my life at that time: ease and happiness. He was simply happy, no matter what was going on. It was a state of being for him, and positive vibes were all around when he came to teach us on Fridays.

Yoga Man's classes were so different from what we practiced while dancing. They weren't focused on strict rules and poses. They were all about the energy and ease of movement. I was such a weirdo for this magic that I went to class every Friday. The poses provided little challenge for me and the other dancers who attended since we moved, jumped, bent, and held tough positions on a regular basis. But while most of the other people couldn't wait for the "nap" at the end of the class, I soaked in the energy of the movement. I had a hunch that the magic wasn't in making the shapes with our bodies; it was in what was happening inside us during this moving meditation.

This experience is what set me on a course to develop Strala Yoga, a movement style that is all about ease and connecting with yourself. It's about focusing on the process rather than stressing about the outcome. It's about tuning in to what feels good for you. It's about letting tension and worry slide away to create space for creativity, passion, improvisation, and joy.

A SHIFT OF FOCUS

Tension is an interesting thing. In a way, it's idolized as something that can help you succeed. If you push hard, fight hard, and work hard, you will get to the top. That's what we're taught. Winning is all about being the one who tries the hardest.

That's how it was for me. I valued my tension. I needed it in an unhealthy way. In my eyes, it was a mark of the hard work, independence, dedication, and effort I needed to achieve. Relaxation wasn't an option. Any approach that involved ease was lazy, unsophisticated, and even irresponsible. It's amazing how I revered my tension, even though, I now realize, it was the main thing holding me back from the life I wanted to lead.

I think a lot of us have this view. We strive. We work. We fight. We follow all the rules, aiming to outdo our colleagues and prove that we're the best. But this also means that we live with continual stress, packing on more tension each day. And when we aren't able to relax, repair, and recover, things go awry.

Yes, stress is helpful when we come face-to-face with a growling dog. Stress gives us a burst of cortisol that spurs us to fight or flee with the best of them. However, if we can't ditch that cortisol and come back to neutral, we begin to break down—both physically and emotionally. We get sick. We get tired. Our creativity and intuition get squashed. We can't go with the flow or be the best versions of ourselves. We simply aren't equipped to deal well with life's everyday challenges.

Let's take a look at a few situations—just so you can see what I mean. Imagine you're in a confrontation with a friend. Or you're in an intense job interview. Or you're trying to master something physical, like a sport or a yoga pose. If you approach any of these situations with tension, things get worse. The confrontation with a friend becomes more frustrating, and you get defensive and lose sight of any input your friend gives. In a job interview, tension leads to an inability to listen or process thoughts clearly. Plus you build nervousness and give off anxious energy. With attempts at physical mastery, you force your body and mind to try to achieve a desired outcome. But this just leads to collected tension that puts your body and mind in a state of panic and stress, which ups your chance of injury.

Let's take the same situations and approach with ease. You take a deep breath to relax, and you listen to your friend. You are able to be in the moment, really hear what's wrong, and improvise in order to come to a meaningful resolution. You take a deep breath to relax before you enter the interview. When your fight-or-flight reaction is under control, you are able to listen and speak logically, clearly, and calmly—plus there's that nice energy you leave behind. With the physical feats, you take a deep breath to relax, tune in to your body, and focus on the process of the movement rather than the goal, and this allows you to accomplish more with less effort.

This movement toward ease in whatever we're doing is what I'm here to talk about.

Whether what we're experiencing is simple or challenging, we can approach it with ease, and when we do, we get further with less effort—often blowing past our goals without even realizing we've already reached them. Why does this happen? Because when we focus on keeping our bodies and minds relaxed and in the moment, we don't look to the future. We don't think about what accomplishing the goal means for the outcome of our lives. By changing our focus to ease, we free up all sorts of energy. Instead of this energy going toward tension and worry, it is free to go in other directions. It can go toward creativity. It can go toward innovation. It can go toward joy and empathy and compassion and so much more. With ease we create the space to choose the direction that is best for us—and the energy to support us in our efforts.

High-level performance of all sorts, mental and physical, is always accomplished with ease. Keep in mind: Ease doesn't mean things are easy. Ease is simply the approach. Ease is the how of what we're doing. And this approach is the secret to awe-inspiring feats accomplished by athletes, great minds, and fantastic artists. What they do seems effortless, but it isn't. It is all about hard work—done from a place of ease.

One beautiful thing about this is that the ability to accomplish more with less effort is available to us all with regular practice. We must practice ease consciously for it to be a regular part of life. Consistently practicing ease of body and mind on your mat will train your body to be incredibly strong and healthy, your mind to be sharp and calm, and your energy levels to be high and vibrant. And this will carry out into every aspect of your life. Soon you will experience ease naturally in that hard conversation with a friend or that intimidating job interview. Practicing ease trains you to move how it feels good and to follow your intuition, which leads to the experience of freedom and having a lot of fun along the way.

When you move with ease through simple and challenging moments alike, you'll blow past your goals in no time. All of a sudden there is so much more room, so much open space, and so much more time to enjoy. With ease, you get happy.

The practice of ease is your golden secret for living a radiant life filled with wonder, strength, surprises, and grace. The practice of ease will put you directly in the moment, where you have room to breathe, create, and enjoy.

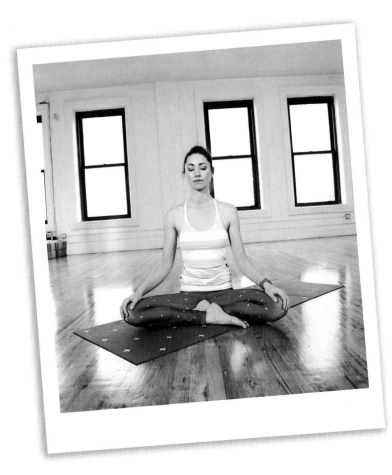

SELF-HELP BREAK

One of the biggest lessons I've learned in my life so far is that change—whether small or large—starts with me. I needed to let go of tension, frustration, and judgment so I could be more loving in the world, which would translate into others feeling more loved and more loving. I could create a ripple effect of love if I could change my own ways.

We all go through tense moments, days, weeks, and even years, but it's never too late to soften, relax, and connect right back inside. With a few simple breaths, we can reconnect to ourselves.

I learned this meditation from my good friend Mallika Chopra. She learned it as a kid from her dad, Deepak Chopra. It's about connecting to what matters most in your life and formulating a clear intent about how you want to be in the world. It's incredibly useful as a daily practice, and it's especially practical when we feel swept up in the stress of life.

So let's take a moment to reconnect in order to shift how you feel. What do you need to let go of? What's holding you back? Freeing yourself from this will help create a shift beyond just you.

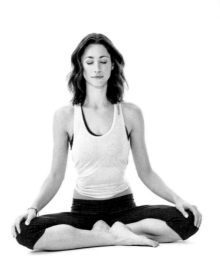

Sit however you are comfortable. Close your eyes and allow your attention to drift inward. Allow yourself to sway side to side and forward and back to find a nice, neutral, balanced place.

Take a big inhale and lift your arms out and up overhead. Press your palms together and bring your thumbs to your heartbeat. Soften here for a moment. Take a big inhale through your nose. Exhale out through your mouth. Twice more just like that. Settle here for a moment.

Take a moment and ask yourself the following questions silently. There is no need to come up with an answer; just ask and allow space for the question to settle with you. Take a few moments in between questions.

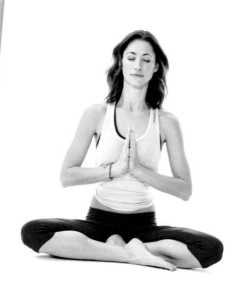

WhO am I?

What dO I want?

HOW can I serve?

When you are ready,
open your eyes and relax your hands on your thighs.

MOVING TOWARD EASE

I know this sounds crazy, but wanting ease isn't people's default—even after they hear about all the amazing things it can do for them. Believing that ease is a good thing takes courage. It takes quite a bit of gusto to discard the idea that working the hardest gets you the most. Shifting to the possibility that an approach of ease might actually be the missing link between where you are now and where you'd like to be isn't simple. It's almost a cruel joke to learn that an approach of ease can help you win—and feel fantastic during the entire process. The great news is the joke is in our favor, and when we choose the approach of ease, we not only achieve what we desire but also feel amazing while we're on the way.

Once you get into this idea that ease is a good thing to have, you have to first find out what it is and how it feels, and then try it on for yourself. Once you start to get to know ease, you can create a life that includes it, which can be an arduous process. I know it was for me.

Back when I was entranced by Yoga Man, I struggled to let go of my tension—it was what got me to where I was. Luckily, Rory, my ballet teacher, saw the confusion I was experiencing. He also saw my interest in yoga, and so one day, he handed me the book *Autobiography of a Yogi*. It was just a gift. At the time, I was actually embarrassed that I was being singled out. In my tension- and worry-filled mind, I thought he might be telling me that I wasn't a very good dancer. But I was also flattered to be noticed for my interest in yoga.

I read the book, which was about the life of Yogananda and his journey bringing yoga to the West. And after reading it, I was inspired. When I learned that there was a Yogananda center in California, I saved up some cash so I could go there over winter break.

During that trip I started to explore different modalities of healing, including Reiki, shiatsu, and other yoga styles. I met a lot of people involved in this world of healing, and, surprisingly, I started to feel disconnected. I was beginning to experience the feeling that Yoga Man radiated, but I was having a difficult time finding like-minded people. Everyone was part of a tradition, a style, or a lineage—and they believed in the power of only their lineage. It wasn't about the magic that lives inside all of us. It was about loyalty to a doctrine. And I just couldn't accept this. In my mind, these traditions were the means to an end; they were the processes that led you to finding your true self. Some processes work for some people and not for others. But the people I met put so much importance on their processes that they seemed to miss the endgame. This world felt just as tense as where I had come from.

The dividedness in this so-called world of love and acceptance made me understand why more people can't access their own magic. I understand how this happens: You have a divine moment while taking part in one tradition, so you dive fully in. Because you never experienced that divine moment with any other practice, you come to the conclusion that those other practices *just. don't. work.* You keep working with the one that resonated, and you reject the others. That's a human tendency. But the obsession with the goodness of the practice often makes us lose sight of the magic.

I felt like this my-way-or-the-highway attitude was keeping people from pursuing yoga and the magic inside them. To many, it remained a secret club, and it was time to bust down the doors.

THE JOY OF HELPING

During this same time, I was starting to realize that becoming a professional dancer wasn't necessarily what I wanted out of life.

I believe that we're all here to help others in some way—and it's always been this way for me. I grew up in the woods of Illinois with an amazing, loving family and lots of open land around me. Like many kids, I loved to run around and play outside. Most of my memories include feeling creative and free and being excited about the limitless possibilities that lay ahead. I loved sitting in nature and practicing a self-taught version of meditation, movement, and connecting to my intuition and the world around me. Tapping into the nature around me felt natural, easy, and fun. When I closed my eyes, I saw bright colors swirling and dancing together, all through me and around me, connecting everything in the most radiant, exciting way. I had a secret conversation with nature, and this was my happy place. It's where I went to revel, enjoy, and dream. Let's just say life was great.

But I also realized that not everyone had it so good. I read about kids around the world who didn't have food to eat or proper homes to live in. In my own life, I saw kids and adults who had all the physical comforts they needed but still suffered from stress and anxiety. I had a burning desire to do whatever I could to help out. I donated my birthday money to the kids who needed food and shelter. I knew it wasn't much, but I had to do something. It was harder to do something for the people who suffered from the more intangible miseries.

I saw teachers get frustrated with students and boil up unnecessarily. I saw people eat too much junk food for comfort and to soothe their stress. I saw my friends' moms hold tension in their bodies because they were worried about so many things. This stress and tension seemed to get worse the longer it went on because people who felt tense and frustrated most of the time were constantly having tense and frustrated interactions. It was a vicious circle. But I also noticed the same type of circle existed for happy people. People who felt mostly happy and free were constantly having happy and free interactions and spreading ease wherever they went.

The energy people gave off was so obvious I felt as if I could almost touch it. I knew that what made me feel good—even if I'd had a crazy day—was connecting back to myself through my nature meditations. This is what put me on the happy circle. And I wanted to help other people feel this. I had no real plan of action, just an inspired feeling of wanting to help.

My desire to help was instilled in me by my parents' reminder—both spoken and by example. They taught my brother and me that helping people and treating everyone equally and with respect, no matter what, were two of the most important things in life. They helped people for no apparent reason, and so that's what I wanted to do. And when I started to help, I felt alive. It didn't matter if I was holding a door, picking up a dropped book, or donating my birthday money to charity, the feeling of helping was amazing. I was hooked on this drug of helping. Yes, the effect of helping someone was nice, but the rush of the feeling was incredible. I wondered why the rush wasn't discussed in lectures of values and kindness. There is something in how we are made up that keeps us feeling great, alive, and vibrant when we help others.

I truly believe that it is our duty to help one another however we can. This is why we are here. When we help one another, we feel connected and good about ourselves. Helping is the key to being able to revel in the magic of who we actually are. Helping others brings out our natural gifts, talents, and strengths. Helping others elevates the individuality of each person and eases desires to show off or prove our worthiness. Helping assumes we all are worthy and works toward a goal of harmony. And it makes us feel pretty awesome.

So, yes, I was hooked on helping, and I couldn't see how dance was helping. Sure, it brought a smile to the people in the audience, but how was it helping in the larger sense? Perhaps this is what made the world of yoga so enchanting. I needed to find the magic that was within me, so I could create a life that spread joy and improved lives.

This desire to help is probably also what fueled some of my frustrations with the yoga culture. People weren't being encouraged to find the light that lives inside them, that inner magic. Many yoga leaders were trying to help people find better health, strength, and stability, but what they lost sight of is that, while we can learn tools from our guides and teachers, the ultimate source is *within*.

The programs that were laid out weren't about the magic; they were about following rules. They were about unbalanced relationships between students and teachers, with a lot of steps required to get to anything supposedly worthwhile.

What had attracted me to this world in the first place seemed so far away. I reflected on my first yoga classes, and I remembered that Yoga Man wasn't like this. He didn't tell us to follow his rules or follow him; he simply shared an approach to tap into the magic and then provided us with the space to own it for ourselves. He influenced by example, just as my parents had.

Now I knew I had an unclear and strange road ahead. I needed to pave a path to help myself connect to the magic, without getting stuck in the rigidity of limiting systems. Discovering my own path of ease and then sharing that with others would be my way of helping.

STARTING ALONG A PATH OF EASE

Even though I wasn't sure that dancing was my future, I moved to New York City to dance. I was lucky in that I also had a lot of opportunities to be in TV commercials and some print campaigns. I loved roaming the city, meeting all kinds of people, and I got myself into random jobs that way. I danced on stilts, choreographed plays, produced documentary films, and a whole host of other interesting things.

It soon got to the point, however, where I had to decide between joining a dance company full time and doing this freelance thing, which gave me a good amount of free time and the ability to pay my rent. I chose the free time and rent. This provided me with some space to figure out what I *actually* wanted to do with my life.

During my free time, I took all kinds of yoga and healing classes. I participated in trainings about healing, philosophy, and loads of different hands-on approaches. I enjoyed dropping in to different yoga communities and floated around to many of them.

I also started to explore my own tension. I have always felt comfortable expressing myself physically, so I investigated dissolving tension through an unlimited physical practice in the safety of my own home. The practice was this: I would move around on my own in what probably looked like a superstrange type of wild woman ceremonial dance. I set no rules for myself. My only goal was to discover.

I took everything I knew, everything I felt, and simply waited to see what would happen. I'd roll around on the floor, on the couch, and on the kitchen counter in an effort to find the tension in my body and mind. I'd try to find out where the tension lived and how I could make it go away. I'd try to find out if this was about effort or relaxation. I'd see what types of movements helped. I'd see where my body ached and where it felt free. Where I was strong and where I was weak. What my body wanted to do once it was in motion.

Through this exploration I realized just how tense I was—in my body, my mind, and my life. I saw how this was affecting me: closing me off and blocking me from accomplishing awesome things. The interconnectedness of mind and body, tension and success, frustration and joy was mind-blowing, scary, and fun.

The biggest thing that happened through my moving exploration was that I started to connect to my intuition. I started to get sensitized to how I felt. And I started to see what was possible. I started to feel free, open, and connected, like I did when I was a kid in nature.

The more I learned, the more excited I became. I continued to explore and roll around like a creature in my apartment. I didn't care if anything more came of this practice. I had no plans, only a quest to feel good and to dissolve my tension.

I carved out some time each day for this wacky exploration. The physicality started to take shape, just like a dance improvisation would mold into choreography. I started to repeat movements and breaths that had a freeing physical and emotional effect. Simple movements that expanded outward and softened back inward were starting to take shape. A routine started to develop and evolve each time I improvised. Without the goal, I had created a self-practice. I felt this was something I wasn't inventing but more remembering. It was coming from a place simultaneously inside me and all around me. I was tapping into something powerful and useful, and I craved more and more.

I wanted other people to feel this too. I knew that most people wouldn't roll around on their floors, so I looked to yoga and meditation. Both help you connect to yourself, just as my crazy-lady dancing did. I shared my interest in feeling good with anyone who would listen. During breaks on shoots, free days, and pretty much whenever, I'd talk about things I thought would help whomever was in front of me. If someone complained about stress, anxiety, back pain, headaches, or sleepless nights, I would do my best to create a little routine to remedy the problem.

I started hearing reports of magic cures from the routines I prescribed— and I was elated. Even stories where people just said the routine made them feel more energetic made me happy. I was getting into the zone of feeling alive again by the simple act of helping. Even better, I started to see a direction for myself. My purpose was starting to show itself through my interest in self-reflection, yoga, movement, and healing.

I also became less angry at people I believed were holding yoga back. I shifted my focus to the power of yoga to help people who wanted to feel better. I had no interest in staking a claim against the systems of yoga; I simply wanted to open up a natural path that could resonate with people. So I started to help people move in ways that felt good to them. I aimed to lead processes clearly and leave my own opinions out.

The approach was working. People started to feel better—they were getting great results and getting really happy. And that's all I wanted. I wasn't interested in being popular, gaining friends, or having admirers. I just wanted to help people. And as I saw people heal and come into themselves, I felt myself coming to life. The more I helped, the happier, more relaxed, and calmer I became. I knew I was starting to spend my time doing something I really loved. Things were getting really fun.

TAKING HELPING FURTHER

Gradually I got a little more structured with my process of helping. I'd go over to people's houses and lead them through a session tailored to their ailments or needs. I loved finding different routines that worked in many kinds of circumstances. What I was learning through working with many people for extended periods of time was a common thread. Tension gets in the way bigtime. I had my own nasty experience with tension taking over my life, and now I could identify it when others were in a tension trap. Like Yoga Man could endure distracted, giggly dancers, I started to find myself immune to people's bad moods and jumpy behavior. I wanted to help reduce the tension, and this yoga stuff approached in an easygoing way was doing the trick.

Soon the word got out. People told their friends about their experiences, and my days became full of one-on-one yoga sessions. At this point, I didn't charge for what I was doing, but people wanted to pay me. I thought it was ridiculous to accept money for doing something I truly loved and that helped people. Luckily, a few people I worked with sat me down, had a mini-intervention, and reminded me that accepting money for this service was not only okay but good. If I did, I could support myself doing what I loved most—and help even more people. I could give up the in-front-of-the-camera work I was doing to pay the bills. I could focus on my happy routine delivery full time.

So that's what I did. I threw on my sweatpants, made a few phone calls, and dived into exploring how to help people with all my time. I was beyond excited and pretty flipped out.

Around that time one of my happy yoga routine clients introduced me to a few publications and suggested I write about my concepts for them. I had all sorts of goofy ideas to bring new people into the world of healing. I made DIY-style videos, blogged, and posted on fun topics like Yoga for Hangovers, Couch Yoga, Yoga for Jocks, and Yoga for Facebook Addicts. The Internet became another platform where I could help people. I figured people would find the posts if they needed the help. Turns out a lot of people needed the help—and doors started to open whenever I had ideas. I started a column for a health magazine and bugged them to publish my first book. After months of being told that yoga is boring and no one wants to read a yoga book, I proved myself with my digital content, and I was able to write and publish a how-to book on yoga. *Slim Calm Sexy Yoga* went better than expected, and doors continued to open.

In the middle of all this momentum, I met my husband, Mike—another agent of ease. I was at a yoga camp as a half joke, trying to get funny footage of my own chocolate withdrawal, life in bunk beds, some lost-in-the-woods stuff, and of course the usual searching-for-the-guru thing.

When Mike and I started talking, it just made sense, and I realized that I was attracting ease into my life in all ways. We got engaged a few months in and married a little over a year later.

Our relationship signified for me another layer of letting go of tension. I now felt comfortable, safe, and at ease. Settling into my new life with Mike opened up space and freedom for me. Layers of tension melted off, and I felt myself coming to the surface and excited to build a structure for helping. I started a free weekly yoga class in Central Park. I sewed a bright-orange flag that said FREE YOGA, and Mike held it up to recruit people for the class. We created a Facebook page. People kept coming back, and we even got in trouble from the park authorities a few times for gathering in too large of a group without a permit. I had regulars and of course loads of drop-ins from people hanging out in the park.

The crew kept building, and soon I felt as if it was time to take this class indoors. Mike and I started a superinformal studio in the living room of our apartment. We had people over every night for class, and the classes quickly became popular and known for being fun, free, open, and direct—and they had good music. People were gaining all kinds of results quickly, from physical strength to emotional release to relief of ailments. It was pretty exciting. We had visitors from out of town who were practicing with my online videos. Journalists stopped by to interview me, even though I had a hard time describing what was going on. The feedback continued to be consistent that the class was different from other yoga classes: it was more fun, more free, less rigid. I started to feel funny about separating myself from other yoga. I didn't want to present something that was less or more, simply something that was useful. I decided I had to deconstruct what I was actually doing and why it felt so good for people.

IT'S ALL ABOUT THE EASE

Soon enough, I realized that the reason the class was so effective was because of its focus on doing what feels good. We were working through the moves while focusing on the process instead of the outcome. In short, we were doing things with ease. I didn't realize it at the time, but I was already teaching people how to do Strala Yoga.

Ease is what Strala is all about. The movements in a Strala class feel very natural, like flowing water. They are fueled by the breath and allow space for the body and mind to accomplish challenges without too much stress.

Everything is interconnected. How we are in our bodies is how we are in our lives. If we can change the way we move, we can change the way we live. Moving like water on the mat—during simple and challenging moments alike—is like selective stress training for life. If you become skilled at approaching hard movements with ease, you will take this attitude to other hard situations in your life. Soon enough you will be on that happy circle. Of course there will still be stress and challenges in life, but what matters most is how you respond and move forward. By creating a life of ease, you will be able to do more with less effort, harness your energy to achieve, and drop tension you don't need along the way.

The Strala practice of moving with ease is designed to put you in the center of the process of self-care. The focus in the practice is on you, moving how it feels great to move, lingering where it feels nice to linger, and giving you space to rest. Strala encourages you to explore the mind-body connection, and it aims to sensitize you to what you truly need. It helps you tap into your intuition through being present and fluid in your movements. By doing this, you not only realize what you need to advance but also turn on your body's natural relaxation response, which helps you recharge, repair, and heal. Combine all of this, and you're in high gear for great results.

The three secrets to Strala lay in drawing on the connection between the breath and the body, tapping into intuition through feeling, and getting in the flow of natural movement. Don't worry; I'll explain each of these fully in the upcoming chapters. For now just know that Strala is an evolution of the practice of yoga and meditation. Time spent practicing soaks into our lives, reflecting lasting results of released tension, heightened creativity, improved connection to self, high confidence, great physical strength, a healthy range of mobility, and an internal state with the space for creativity and joy. Simply, it leaves you feeling fantastic from the inside out.

THE EASE EXPERIMENT

Let's do a simple, fun experiment. Wherever you are, tense up your whole body. Clench your muscles, make tight fists, and furrow your brow. Now try to get up and walk across the room, keeping the tension intact.

How did that go?

Okay, I know it probably felt a little silly and maybe even a bit stressful. Many people who do this feel their minds tensing in addition to their bodies. They feel frustration building, anxiety rising, and stress levels skyrocketing—just from a short tense walk.

Okay. Let's shake it off and relax. We'll reset the mood.

Stay standing and take a big inhale and lift your arms out and up. Take a long exhale and soften your arms down by your sides. Take a moment here for a few more deep breaths. Now go for that same walk across the room.

Pretty big difference, isn't it? Of course, this is a dramatic exercise, but it reveals just how much our tension can get in the way of every move we make.

NATURE'S EASE

As humans we have the ability to choose how we live, which is obviously fantastic for developing our lives, but it can be harmful if we forget our natural state—a state of ease. Whenever I need to do something more to reconnect to my intuition and my own sense of ease, I return to nature.

Nature is an incredible system that balances itself, shifting without hesitation, bending with the breeze, washing over the shore under the careful direction of the moon, growing and resting with the rise and set of the sun. Our fantastic ecosystem is full of checks and balances that keep everything fluid and working for the greater good. It exists in a state of free-flowing ease and harmony—just as we are supposed to.

When we use nature as a guide, we are reminded to apply wisdom, freedom, movement, and beauty to our lives. We remember to soften into the flow of the elements around us. By finding the ease displayed by nature, our tension dissolves, our minds sharpen and clear, and our bodies strengthen and find balance.

But it's easy to fall into feeling separate from nature in our task- and success-oriented lives. That feeling of separation takes us away from the reality that we are nature, and that we are connected to the things around us. We forget that we are part of an ecosystem, and we test our limits of how unnatural we can be and still thrive. We pile on the work, take on gobs of stress, and work ourselves up with expectations and frustrations. We get out of balance and sick, and something eventually breaks. We try to control everything. We refuse to stop, slow down, rest, and care for ourselves. It's completely unnatural.

Imagine if a tree refused to let a bird build a home on one of its branches because it felt slighted, or refused to let the wind blow its leaves because it was in a grumpy mood. That silly picture of moody nature isn't so far off what we do to ourselves in our daily lives. We wind ourselves up so much and create tension that doesn't need to be there. We lose the connection to who we truly are—stamping out our intuition and leaning on the rules that other people have made.

We can learn loads about how we work by observing nature. When we practice yoga with nature in mind and absorb the elements of who we are as we flow, we are reminded that ease is the winning approach. The practice of coming back to the breath, allowing the body to move fueled by the breath, and allowing space for the mind to be calm and expand shows us that even when we veer toward a reaction of tension, ease is always waiting for us to settle right back in. Ease is the practice that reminds us who we are. We aren't stressed-out, frustrated people. When we have our tense moments, we can remember that they are only moments. We can always choose ease. Once we understand how ease works, we hopefully continue to make the choice.

FINDING YOUR HEART

At the beginning and end of each Strala class, we do this exercise, which has a similar benefit to going out into nature. Connecting to our heartbeat is a tangible way to sensitize ourselves to what is happening with us in the moment and guiding ourselves to a calm, harmonious, energized state.

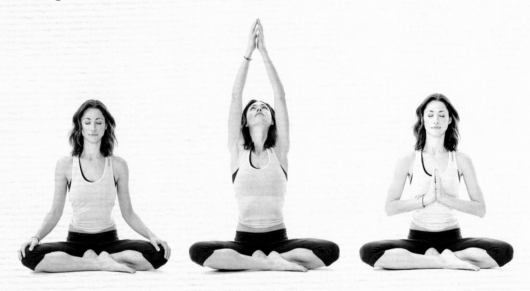

Sit comfortably, wherever you are. It can be in a chair, on the couch, or on the floor, however you are easy in your body. Close your eyes and take a few deep breaths. Take a big inhale and lift your arms out and up overhead. Press your palms together and bring your thumbs right to your heartbeat. Settle here for a moment. See if you can feel your heart pumping for you. Take a big inhale through your nose. Long exhale out through your mouth. Twice more just like that. Big inhale through your nose. Long exhale out through your mouth. One more time. Big inhale through your nose. Long exhale out through your mouth. Settle here for a moment. When you are ready, open your eyes and relax your arms at your sides.

TAKING STRALA FORMAL

Once I figured out why this type of yoga was so powerful, I decided to officially set up shop. I needed a name for the studio, so Mike and I wrote words that were inspiring and captured the spirit of the feeling people got from practice. A few words kept coming up. *Strength. Balance. Awareness.* We mushed the words together and invented a new word: *Strala.* It sounded cool to both of us, so we went with it. I found out later, after a few Swedish people visited and a Swedish newspaper wrote a story on the studio that we didn't actually make up this word. It exists in Swedish (but with a circle above the first *a*: *Stråla*), and it means to radiate light. It also means to smile broadly, which is just awesome.

We set up the studio downtown in New York City and started having a ton of fun all the time. People from around the world would hear about us and come by for a class when they were visiting New York. Many of them had been moving with ease along with the videos and posts I made online, which meant that they already had cool stories of transformation. It was awesome to see the reach of digital media, but it was even more fun to see how the concept of ease was helping people. I was humbled, and I knew these people were helping themselves. I was simply sharing an approach that had helped me.

After years of leading classes that were simply called "yoga" and seeing the amazing results that came from it, I was ready to embrace Strala as its own thing. It was different and special. Even longtime yoga practitioners and instructors from other types of studios got on the bandwagon. They started implementing elements of Strala into their own practices and teachings. They chose to replace the rigidity of yoga with the experience of freedom. Following someone else's rules was replaced with discovering and exploring your own. Strala was undeniably invigorating, so we decided to make its instruction a bit more formal. We started to train people to teach in the Strala way so they could inspire more people to figure out what made them feel healthy and alive.

We wanted a more specific description for our instructors than the word *teacher*, since the class is about sharing the process. *Teacher* created a problem of superiority and separateness and a warped relationship to the student. We all are on this journey together, no matter what our role is, finding our way into what we already have, on a quest to uncover our magic that is resting inside, waiting for us to tap in. So we decided to use the word *guide*. Strala guides do the important job of keeping people safe and delivering a clear process to help them connect back to themselves. The main job of the guide is to stay out of the way, providing help only when it is needed. Just like when you climb a mountain: The guide shows you where to step, how to avoid the crevasse, when to rest, and things like that. The guide is climbing with you, has experience with the mountain, and keeps you safe. Strala guides are interested in achieving with ease, and empowering people to find their own magic.

Every guide is unique and brings something special and awesome to his or her class. I'm proud of our individuality and freedom of expression in guiding to a common goal rather than forcing guides to keep with a specific form. We have a common language of easygoing movement and a structure with loads of freedom inside so you can move how it feels good to you.

These days, and probably until I'm done here on Earth, you will find me shuffling around the studio, leading classes, working with guides, and hanging out with the awesome community. We have guides leading classes in partner studios and clubs around the world, spreading this ease and radiating positive vibes.

I like to describe Strala as its own universe where we have a goal of connecting to the self, and there are certain elements that go into the soup of orchestrating that experience. In other universes of yoga, there are other goals and other elements. I don't intend to imply that one universe is better than the other, simply that there are differences that make sense in each universe. In Strala the trees are purple (or whatever color you want them to be), the sky is clear, and the birds are guided by a big sense of ease. The goal of Strala Yoga is to create strength and balance in the body, and a calm, easy, focused mind. The practice is designed to be fun, freeing, and enjoyable. You'll be encouraged to move with your breath, linger where it feels nice to linger, and explore what feels great for you. The movements are designed to open, expand, create space, and move you into yourself. I'm thrilled to share this practice with you, and I encourage you to share a little more ease and fun with those around you who need it most. You will change some lives for the better and help all of us out along the way.

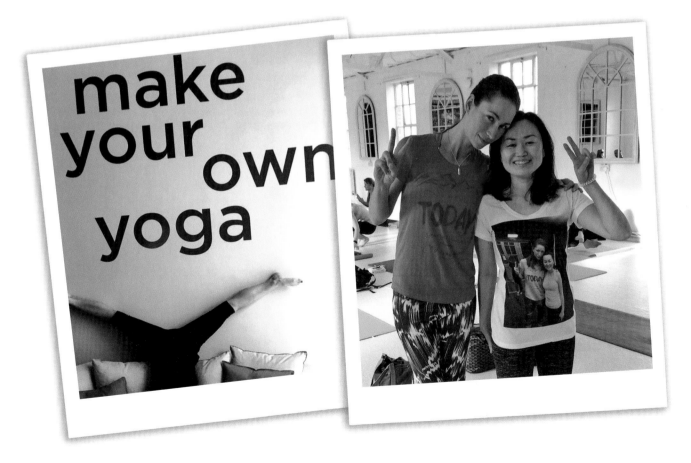

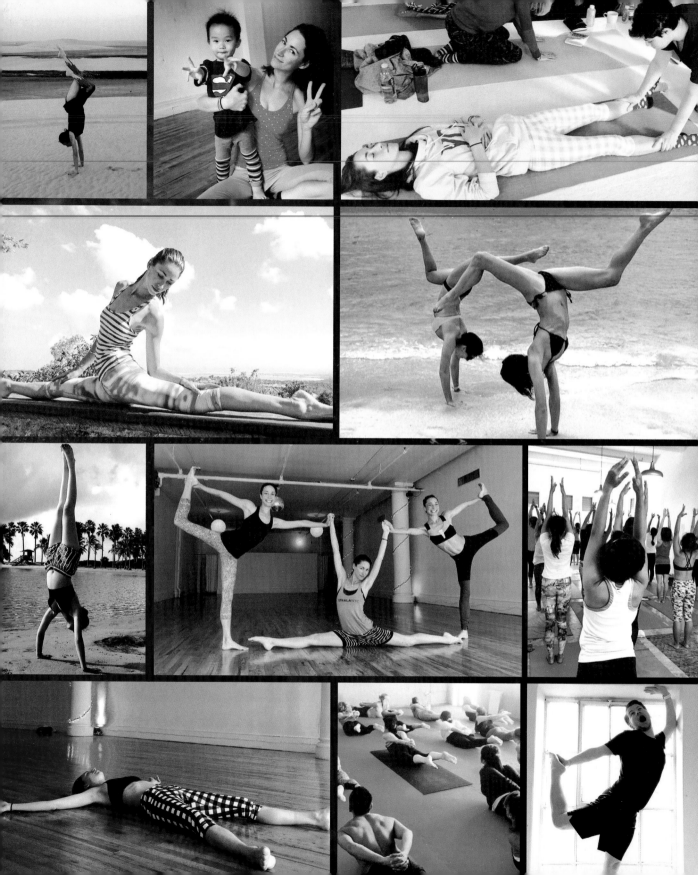

CHAPTER 2

CREATE SPACE

the breath-body connection

The first secret of moving with ease; getting more done with less effort; cultivating lasting strength, balance, and awareness; and feeling fantastic is actually something we do all day long. We do it without thinking, without effort, without planning. It's our most undervalued, underutilized, natural, sustainable, renewable resource. When we deepen it, we energize, strengthen, and lift our bodies. When we fill up with it, we focus and calm our minds.

When we rest our attention on it, we slide into an awesome state of safety, remembrance, and gratitude. And when we cultivate a regular practice of paying attention to it, we strengthen our ability to regulate, repair, restore, and recover.

I'm sure you've guessed by now that I'm talking about the breath. The breath can fuel the body to move like water. And paying attention to your breath creates a fluid approach to movement that puts you right in the flow of the process. It taps you into your intuition, creativity, and focus. It shifts you into cultivating superhuman strength, a healthy range of motion, and radiant health. Focusing on the breath settles you into the relaxation response, where you are able to hit the reset button, strengthen immunity, and switch on your body's ability to relax, restore, heal, and recover.

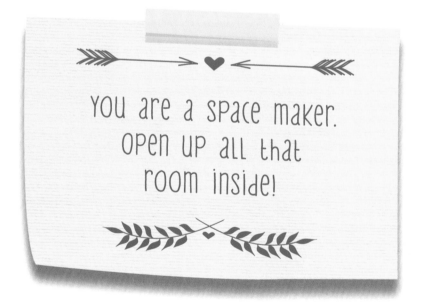

You are a space maker.
Open up all that
room inside!

Our breath is the foundation for how we experience our lives. When we are relaxed, we naturally breathe deeply, our bodies soften, and our minds are calm. When we are stressed, we breathe short and fast, our bodies stiffen, and our minds are frazzled. When we are relaxed, we can see more of a big picture.

We have an optimistic view of our lives. We feel happy and content. When we are stressed, we see a distorted, narrow view of our lives. We feel fried and distracted. The breath is an amazing tool that we can use to come back to relaxation and navigate our lives with grace and ease. And when we use it consciously to accompany our movements, it becomes a power source that will take us through simple and challenging moves alike.

A SIMPLE BREATH

Before we dive more deeply into our study of the breath, let's try a super-simple experiment. Close your eyes and simply bring your attention to your breath. Is it short, fast, long, or deep? Something else? Just watch it as it comes in and rolls out. Notice the space between your breaths. If you notice your attention wandering away from your breath, see if you can guide it right back. Become an easy observer of what is happening, just as you are when you lie on the grass on a warm sunny day and watch the clouds drift by in the sky. Stay with this for a few more moments, and when you are ready, gently open your eyes.

It's pretty cool, right? While you may simply feel a little more relaxed and open after this experiment, there's so much more that can come from paying attention to the breath. The power of a whole universe exists right there inside you. Your own personal world of limitless possibilities. A well of answers, beauty, relaxation, and wonder. A connection to everything around and a grounding of self, right inside. All the comforts of safety and home, right there waiting. The breath is our ultimate nourishment, and when we start to pay attention to it, we begin to realize we can do all sorts of awesome things and enjoy the ride along the way.

You can do this easy practice anytime, anywhere. The simple act of observation creates space that helps us gain perspective, slow down scattered or racing thoughts, and tap into our creativity, intuition, and purpose.

Just imagine what would happen if you made a regular practice of paying attention to the breath.

When I started a morning breath practice, a lot of things shifted besides my breathing. It wasn't anything much at first, but everything began to unfold in the direction of what I wanted to happen. I was experiencing flow state. (Still am, thankfully!) Doors were starting to open easily, I was in the right place at the right time more often, and I was enjoying the situations and moments of my life a lot more. Synchronicities started to happen often. For example, when my first book was getting ready to go to print, I needed a cover blurb from someone awesome. My publisher asked me who that awesome person would be, and, without thinking, I blurted out, "Deepak Chopra! He's awesome, and he probably would like what I do." The only problem was that I had never met Deepak, so getting an endorsement might be tough. But the next day I got an

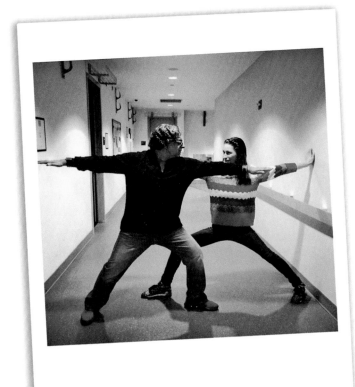

e-mail asking me to teach a yoga class for an event Deepak would be speaking at. Of course I said yes! At the event, Deepak asked me to be part of an iPhone app idea he had for yoga. We went on to collaborate on many projects and became friends over the years. Oh, and he so graciously did that blurb for me.

Other great things happened too. It was just synchronicities. The way I felt improved dramatically. I felt connected with the world around me. I was able to help people I was working with one-on-one even more effectively.

There is a sweet spot that opens up when we allow 10 to 20 minutes each morning to sit and connect with our breath. The relaxation and space we feel during our breathing meditations color the rest of our days. It starts us off on a good foot, which means we're able to deal with the everyday frustrations that rear their ugly heads. Not to mention the other benefits that come from this practice: a deeper connection to ourselves, those around us, and our lives' purposes; improved immunity, health, and overall well-being; sharpened focus; enhanced creativity; improved sleep and energy—the list goes on and on. I would wager that if you can think of something in your life that you would like to improve, a morning breathing practice will help.

THE FIRST ELEMENT OF EASE

The breath-body connection is the main ingredient to moving with ease. When we start to move with ease, we naturally begin to breathe deeper. But we can turn this on its head, consciously choosing to breathe more deeply. By doing this, we can employ our breath to fuel our movement, so our body simply goes along for the ride. Within the system of Strala, this is the first thing we focus on.

The breath has the ability to sensitize us to how we feel, allowing our relaxation response to work for us and heal imbalances efficiently and naturally. The breath can lift, soften, move, and power our bodies and minds any direction we'd like to go, while taking the labor-intensive pressure off so we can enjoy the ride. We have a lot of fun when we move with the breath. When we move absent the breath, we can probably still accomplish most tasks, but they are harder than they need to be and they're a lot less fun. Our ever-present breath is often taken for granted and ignored, but when we bring attention to our breath, we can use it to achieve so much more with ease, leaving space for mental clarity, creativity, and restoration along the way.

A BREATHING EXPERIMENT

Let's try a fun experiment to see how much we can improve our experience with our breath in a supersimple way. Stay where you are right now; whether you are standing, sitting, or lying down, it doesn't matter. Lift your right arm. Lower your right arm. Lift your left arm. Lower your left arm. Lift both arms. Lower both arms.

Okay, that wasn't too complicated, I know. For most of us, that's a pretty easy exercise that doesn't require a lot of strength or effort. We can probably lift our arms without much concentration. It's a simple movement.

Now let's try it again with the breath. Take a moment and close your eyes. Rest your attention a little deeper inward. Take a big inhale and fill up. Take a long exhale and relax. Take a big inhale and lift your right arm up. Exhale and soften it down. Take a big inhale and float your left arm up. Easy exhale and rest it down. Take a huge inhale and lift both arms up. Soft exhale and relax your arms down by your sides.

How did that go? Probably a little more enjoyable, a little more spacious, and a little more graceful of a feeling, right?

In the Strala classes, we use the breath to fuel movement. You don't have to worry or think about anything. We take care of it for you by guiding it in the instruction. Not every inhale and exhale is said or guided, but when the body is doing something where the breath can help, the breath is front and center. Inhales do all the heavy lifting. Exhales do all the softening. A down dog split often comes along with a big inhale to help you lift the leg up and back. Next obviously comes an exhale, but depending on what move follows your down dog split, we may or may not tell you to breathe. You're naturally going to breathe out, so we only note it if it will help the movement. If I cued your every movement with either an inhale or an exhale, you might throw your yoga mat at me five minutes into the class. Over the years, through a lot of mistakes mostly, we've learned when it is effective to guide the breath and when it is effective to leave people alone to feel.

The other instance when I note how to breathe is in moments where we would stay for a few breaths in a pose or a movement. The breath gives life to the pose, so it makes sense to call it a movement. In child's pose, for example, I would remind you to hang for a few big, deep breaths. I remind you to relax and breathe by guiding you with something to do. Guiding the open space of breathing instead of telling you when to inhale and exhale in child's pose is a purposeful instruction to create a sense of ease and freedom in the moment. If I told you to inhale and exhale five times on my cue, you would have a higher chance of either getting agitated with me or buying into my logic that it is a good idea to only inhale and exhale when I say so. Either way it's not very much fun.

Powering movement and encouraging spacious rest are both aims of focusing on the breath. And when we do this, something awesome happens. The body works and moves for you. It clicks into efficiency mode. Worries subside, movements become smooth, and space opens up for the mind to be reflective and enter a meditative state. When we are easy in our bodies and minds as we move, we can enter into a moving meditation. When we move absent the breath, we spend most of our mental power on the task of moving.

Another cool thing that happens is that paying attention to the breath changes our perception of time. When we move without the breath front and center, time seems to drag on. Movements become a little stiff, labored, and we start to locate our attention in our minds. We begin to think about when the pose will end, how much longer the class is, or even what we'll have for dinner. When we move with the breath as the fuel, we settle right into a "flow state" where we feel amazing. Movements happen easily, we are out of our heads, and we enjoy it and have fun. We don't notice the time passing.

Here are a few fun ways to visualize the breath-body connection:

☆ **Every inhale opens a door. Every exhale walks you right through.**

☆ **Each inhale creates space. Each exhale moves you into the space.**

☆ **Each inhale strengthens. Each exhale softens.**

☆ **Every inhale fills you up. Every exhale settles.**

☆ **The inhale lifts and does the work for you. The exhale softens you right in.**

When you employ the breath-body connection in your yoga practice, your movements become fun, easy, and circular. Your breath and body move together, putting you in an oceanic rhythm. The waves roll in and drift out. You lift and soften as you move. You rise and settle as you glide. You are putting in the effort. Your breath is fueling the work for you.

Think back for a moment to that simple experiment—the one where you lifted your arms with and without your breath. While that movement took barely any work, it should have felt different with the breath. But imagine when things really get cooking and you're doing a hard move. Imagine rocking forward and back in a handstand. This could be exciting or terrifying, depending on how you feel about handstands. With the breath, you can find ease in your effort; without the breath, a handstand is purely effort. By focusing on the breath, you are focusing on the process of doing the handstand—not simply the goal. And this is a key factor with Strala—it's about the process, not the goal.

WHAT ABOUT THE WORKOUT?

Working and moving with the breath instead of pushing through with muscular force is a big change for the way many people work. If you're like a lot of folks who come to Strala classes, moving with ease may bring a couple of questions to mind. Specifically: "Where is the workout in this easy way of moving?" and "How am I working hard if I am not clenching and flexing my muscles while I move?" You have no idea how many times people have questioned whether a workout focused on ease is *actually* a workout.

My answer to them is: "Yes! Of course it's a workout. And a good one."

Think about lions out in the wilderness. They don't clench their muscles when they run and climb and chase. They simply go. They move naturally, and they accomplish their goals. They're also fit and don't have to go to a gym to stay that way.

The movements in the Strala vocabulary, which we'll cover later, combined with the breath-body connection, are designed to cultivate a natural, animal-like, efficient body and a calm, focused mind. Unlike a lot of traditional yoga classes where you perform a pose, break the pose, and then perform another pose, Strala classes move a whole lot. There are no poses, only movements, and the whole class becomes one easy movement happening with the breath.

Using the breath as your fuel, you are able to accomplish much more with your body than if you simply forced your way through the routine, so you actually get more of a workout. Your muscles are able to work efficiently when you aren't flexing and clenching them.

We accomplish a lot in one class. You move your body in every way it can naturally move. You balance on two feet, one foot, two hands, and one hand. You move from your center and lift your own body weight. People who practice Strala regularly are incredibly fit, strong, and healthy. Some use Strala as a successful mental and physical cross-training for other athletic endeavors. Some use Strala as their main form of fitness. Any way you use Strala, it is a fantastic workout.

LET'S PRACTICE!

All right! I think you're ready to move a bit more so you can fully experience the power of the breath-body connection. The following routine is pretty simple. I'm going to take you through it twice: once without the breath cues and once with them.

The first round will be without the cues; I'll guide movement only. Of course, you'll still be breathing—it simply won't be intentional breathing. In the second round, I will guide you through the same routine with the breath as your fuel. Take note of any differences in how you feel.

The goal here is to notice how your body feels when you add different elements. I hope this routine will help you experience how useful your breath can be in accomplishing movement, creating space in your body and mind, and getting you in the flow.

SIMPLE MOVEMENT ROUTINE

MOVING WITHOUT THE BREATH

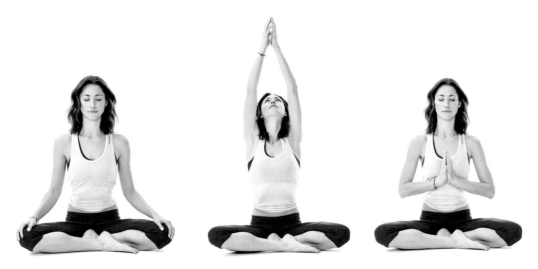

Sit comfortably. Lift your arms up. Press your palms together.
Bring your thumbs to your heartbeat. Inhale through your nose.
Exhale out through your mouth. Twice more like that. Inhale through
your nose. Exhale through your mouth. Inhale through your nose.
Exhale through your mouth. Relax your hands on your thighs.

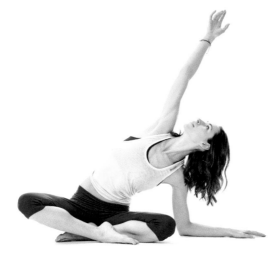

Press your right hand on the
ground to your side. Bend your
torso to the side. Soften your
elbow, resting your forearm on
the ground. Stay here for a few
moments. Bring your torso up
through the center and do the
same on the other side.

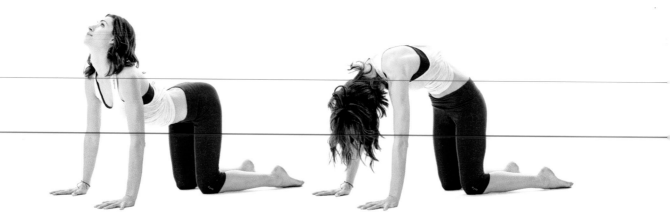

Come onto all fours. Drop your belly, arch your back, and look up.
Round your back and look down. Repeat this three times.

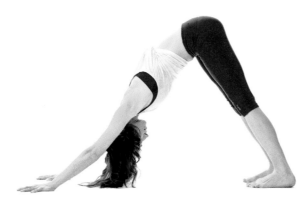

Tuck your toes and lift your hips
up and back to down dog.

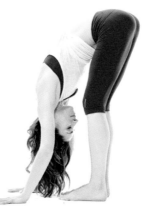

Walk your feet up to your hands
and fold your torso over your legs.

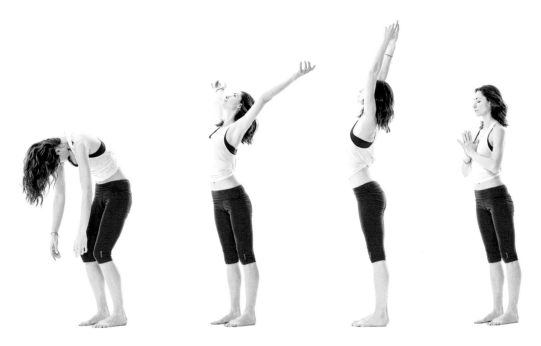

Roll your torso up to standing. Lift your arms up and look up. Exhale and press your palms together and bring your thumbs to your heartbeat.

Okay, how did that feel? Since I'm not there with you right now I'll take a guess and see if we're on the same page. I'm guessing it went okay, but nothing too exciting happened. It might have felt a little wonky even, a bit rigid possibly, and maybe even challenging. Maybe you felt a little stuck in each pose, and the goal was to get through the poses until the routine was over. Usually this is the feedback when I lead this exercise with groups. Interestingly a lot of people also report that they feel as though they are being told what to do and even feel inadequate at times. People consistently say this type of guidance puts the instructor in charge and the person doing the routine feels close to being bossed around. It can feel boring, as well, or more close to an exercise routine where we are waiting for it to be finished so we can relax. Maybe you felt none of this, and it felt okay. That's totally fine too. That happens.

Take a moment to reflect on how this routine felt to you. If you want, write it down. When you're ready, let's try this again with the breath-body connection and see if you feel any difference.

MOVING FUELED WITH THE BREATH

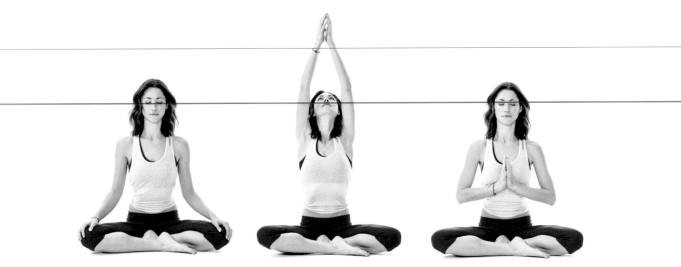

Sit comfortably. Allow your body to move a bit easy with your breath to find a nice, neutral place. Take a few breaths and settle here for a moment. Take a big inhale and lift your arms up. Press your palms together. Bring your thumbs to your heartbeat. Soften here for a moment. Take a big inhale through your nose. Long exhale out through your mouth. Twice more like that. Big inhale through your nose. Easy exhale through your mouth. Last time, deep inhale through your nose. Long exhale through your mouth. Relax your hands on your thighs and soften here for a moment.

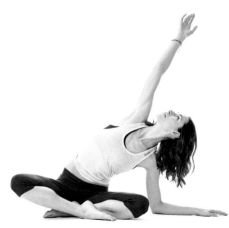

Staying soft and easy, tip over to your right side, pressing your right hand and forearm on the ground. Reach your opposite arm overhead and hang here for a few long, deep breaths. Bring your torso up through the center and go for the other side.

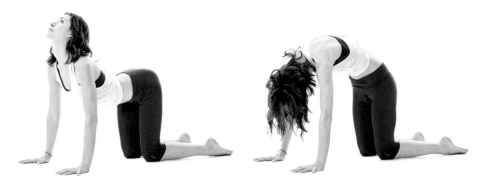

Come onto all fours easy with your breath. Take a big inhale, dropping your belly, arching your back, and looking up. Exhale and round your back and look down. Roll through this motion softly with your breath three times.

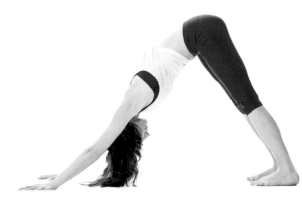

Tuck your toes, take a big inhale, and lift your hips up and back to down dog.

Walk your hands and relax your torso gently over your legs.

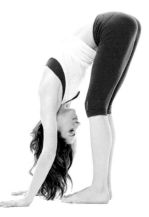

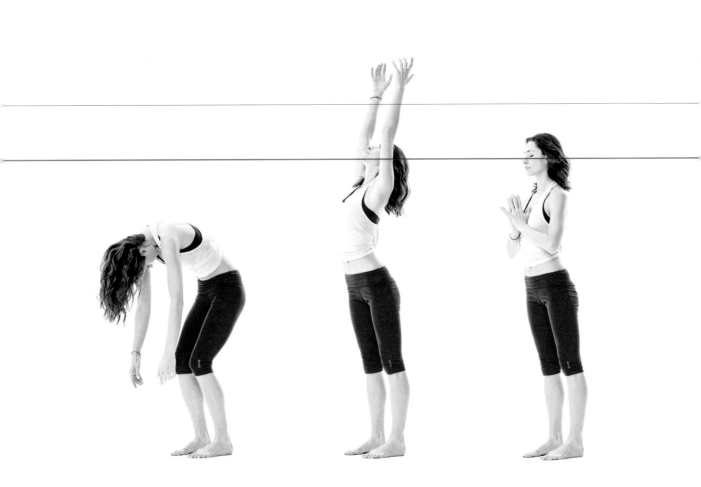

Roll your torso up to standing.
Take a big inhale and lift your arms up, out, and up.
Exhale and press your palms together and bring
your thumbs to your heartbeat.

How did that feel? You probably experienced how the breath has a big capability to soften and fuel the movement, making it easier and lighter. The breath takes the labor and heavy lifting out of the body and allows us to go along for the ride of the movement. Without the breath, movement becomes tougher than it needs to be, and that tension trickles right into the mind and closes in our sense of space and ease.

A BIT OF A CHALLENGE

If you're up for it, here is a routine for you that includes a bit more movement to really get your entire body moving with your breath. Some of these moves are pretty tough, so do what you can. Feel free to skip a move or stop the routine if there is something out of your reach. We'll do the same thing we did last time: first time through without breath cues, second time with them. Doing both of these variations will really help you see just how powerful the breath can be. Unlike the last routine, you may not be able to do some of the poses when you're moving without the breath, but once you bring the breath in, you may complete them or you'll come a heck of a lot closer.

MOVING WITHOUT THE BREATH

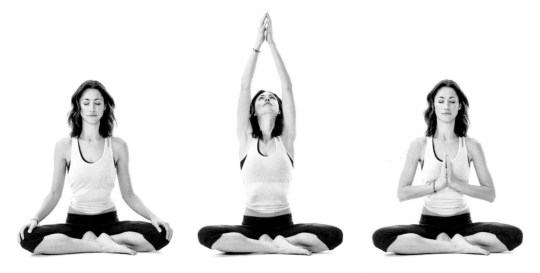

Sit comfortably. Lift your arms up. Press your palms together. Bring your thumbs to your heartbeat. Inhale through your nose. Exhale out through your mouth. Twice more like that. Inhale through your nose. Exhale through your mouth. Inhale through your nose. Exhale through your mouth. Relax your hands on your thighs.

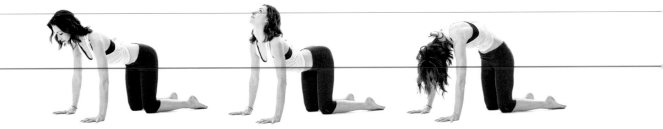

Come onto all fours. Drop your belly, arch your back, and look up.
Round your back and look down. Repeat three times.

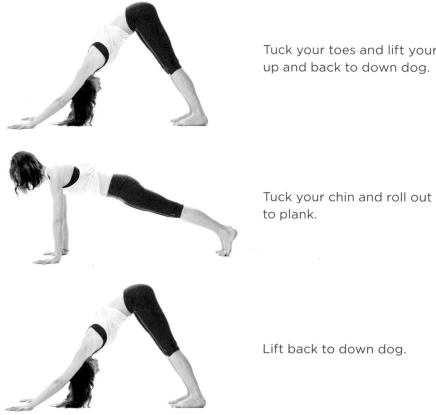

Tuck your toes and lift your hips
up and back to down dog.

Tuck your chin and roll out
to plank.

Lift back to down dog.

Tuck your chin and roll out to plank.

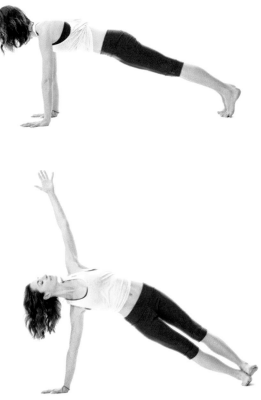

Shift your weight onto your right hand and the outside edge of your right foot and open your body into a side plank facing your left side. If you want some more stability, soften your right shin to the ground for support.

Come back into plank.

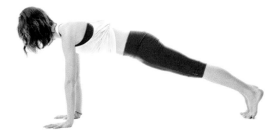

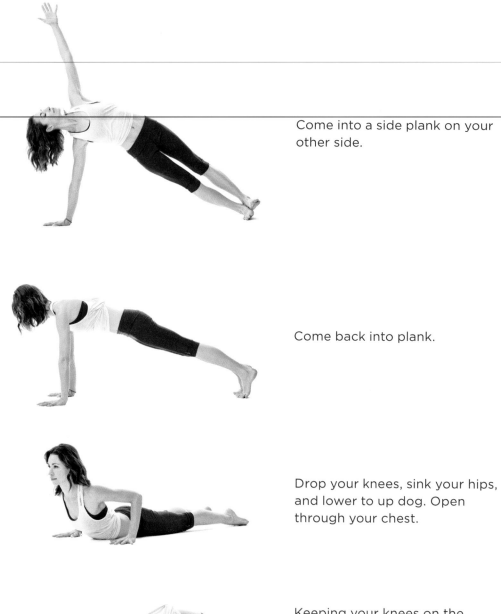

Come into a side plank on your other side.

Come back into plank.

Drop your knees, sink your hips, and lower to up dog. Open through your chest.

Keeping your knees on the ground, shift your hips to your heels, and relax your torso on the ground into child's pose.

Come back onto all fours, tuck your toes, and lift up and back into down dog.

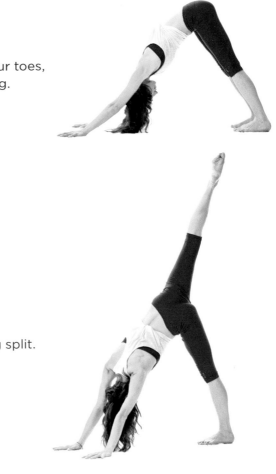

Lift your right leg up to down dog split.

Step your foot through to low lunge.

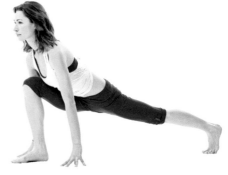

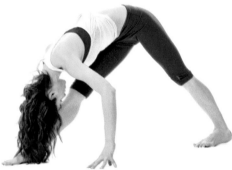

Lower your back knee down.
Open up your chest.
Lift your arms up.

Press your fingertips to the ground.
Tuck your back toes, lift your hips
up, and relax your torso over your
front leg.

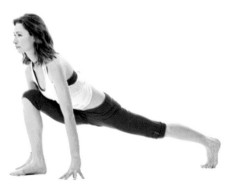

Sink your hips to your low lunge.

Lift up into a high lunge. Lift your hips and lift your arms overhead.

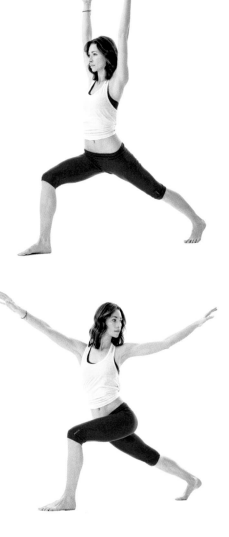

Twist to your front leg and open your arms out to your sides.

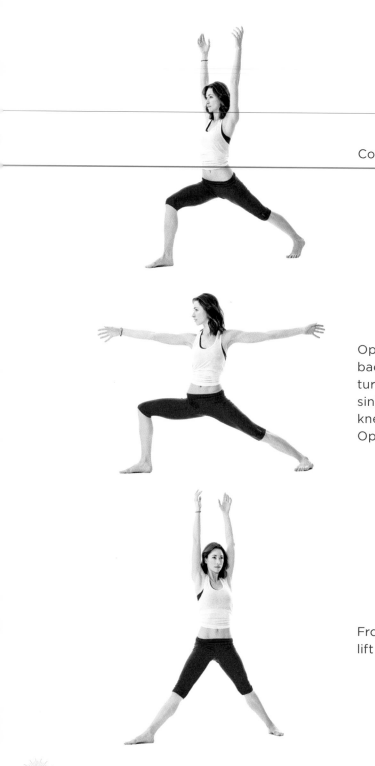

Come back into high lunge.

Open into warrior 2. Ground your
back heel down, toes slightly
turned toward your front foot, and
sink your hips low so your front
knee comes over your front foot.
Open your arms out to your sides.

From warrior 2 lift your hips and
lift your arms up over your head.

Sink back into warrior 2.

Tip your torso back into reverse warrior. Slide your back hand down your back leg, and extend your front arm and torso up and back over your head.

Tip your torso up and over into your extended side angle. Press your top forearm on your front thigh, arc your back arm up and over your head, and roll your torso open.

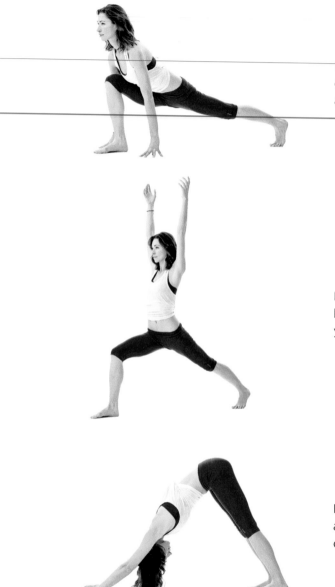

Bring your fingertips to the ground
on either side of your front foot
and sink your hips into low lunge.

Lift up into high lunge. Lift your
hips and lift your arms up and over
your head.

Press your palms into the ground
and make your way back to down
dog.

Repeat on the other side.

MOVING FUELED WITH THE BREATH

Here we go again, using the breath to our advantage.

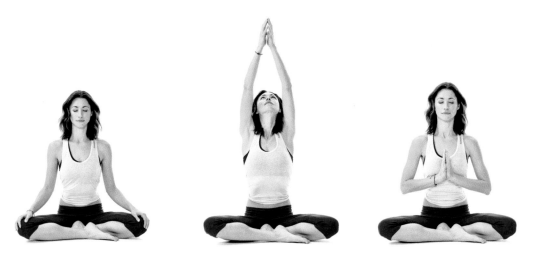

Sit comfortably. Settle in for a moment. Take a big inhale and lift your arms up. Press your palms together. Bring your thumbs to your heartbeat. Soften here for a moment. Take a big inhale through your nose. Long exhale out through your mouth. Twice more like that. Big inhale through your nose. Easy exhale through your mouth. One more time, big inhale through your nose. Long exhale through your mouth. Relax your hands on your thighs.

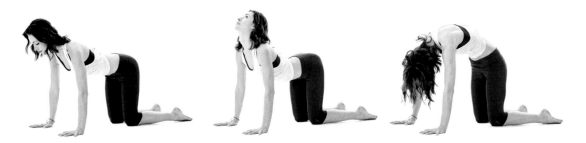

Come onto all fours. Take a big inhale, drop your belly, arch your back, and look up. Exhale, round your back, and look inward. Move through this a few times, easy with your breath.

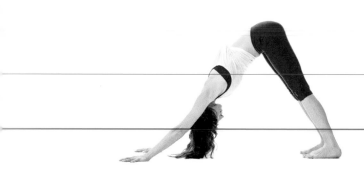

Tuck your toes, take a big inhale, and lift your hips up and back into down dog.

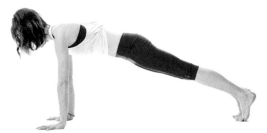

Tuck your chin and roll out to plank.

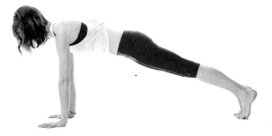

Take a big inhale and lift up and back to down dog.

Tuck your chin and roll out to plank.

Shift your weight onto your right hand and the outside edge of your right foot. Take a big inhale and open your body into a side plank facing your left side. If you want some more stability, soften your right shin to the ground for support.

Come back into plank.

Come into a side plank on your other side. Take a big inhale and open up here.

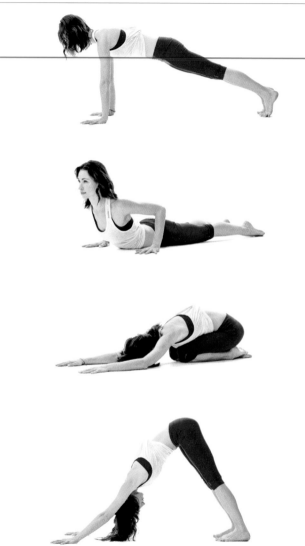

Come back into plank.

Drop your knees, sink your hips, and lower to up dog. Open through your chest, moving along easy with your breath.

Keeping your knees on the ground, shift your hips to your heels and relax your torso on the ground into child's pose. Hang here for a few big, deep breaths.

Come back onto all fours, tuck your toes, take a big inhale, and lift your hips up and back into down dog.

Take a big inhale, and lift your
right leg up to down dog split.

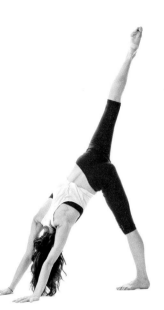

Step your foot through to
low lunge.

Lower your back knee down. Open up your chest easy
with your breath. Take a big inhale and lift your arms up.

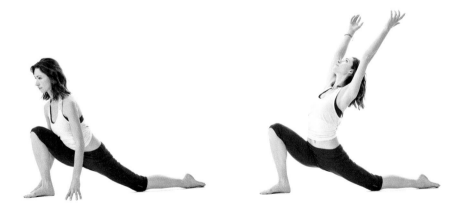

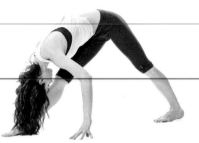

Press your fingertips to the ground. Tuck your back toes, take a big inhale, lift your hips up, and relax your torso over your front leg.

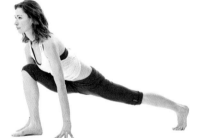

Sink your hips to low lunge.

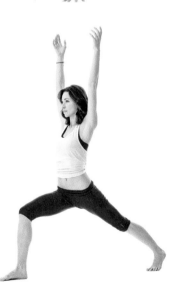

Push down through your legs, take a big inhale, and lift up into high lunge. Lift your hips and lift your arms overhead.

Exhale and twist toward your front leg, and open your arms out to your sides.

Big inhale and come back into high lunge.

Easy exhale and open into warrior 2. Ground your back heel down, toes slightly turned toward your front foot, and sink your hips low so your front knee comes over your front foot. Open your arms out to your sides. Settle in here for a moment.

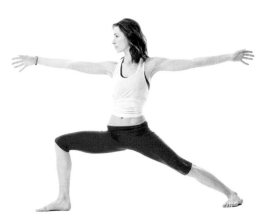

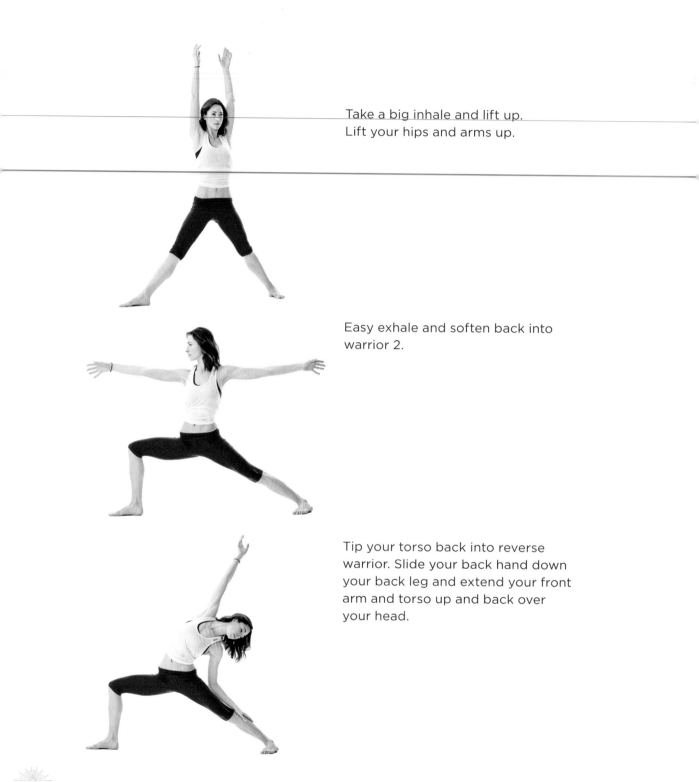

Take a big inhale and lift up.
Lift your hips and arms up.

Easy exhale and soften back into
warrior 2.

Tip your torso back into reverse
warrior. Slide your back hand down
your back leg and extend your front
arm and torso up and back over
your head.

Tip your torso up and over into your extended side angle. Press your top forearm on your front thigh, arc your back arm up and over your head, and roll your torso open.

Bring your fingertips to the ground on either side of your front foot and sink your hips into low lunge.

Push down through your legs, take a big inhale, and lift up into high lunge. Lift your hips and lift your arms up and over your head.

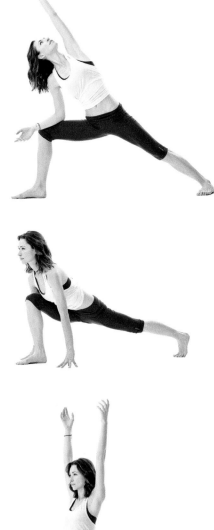

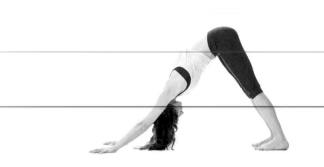

Exhale right back down to the ground, plant your palms, and make your way back to down dog.

Repeat on the other side.

How did that feel? Notice any difference? Most people do. Just like in the Simple Movement routine, the majority of folks report that the difference with the breath is massive. More spacious, lighter, freer, and more fun! The movements feel physically roomier and mentally easier with the breath as the fuel. Time flies by, and the experience feels fun and free. You are a space maker, and the path in is your breath.

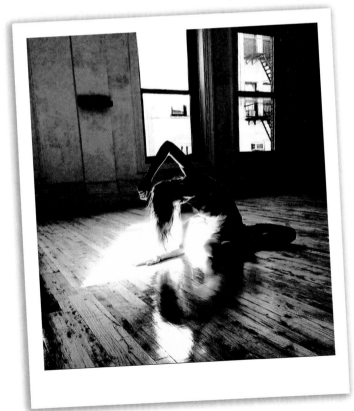

This idea of creating space physically and mentally becomes a reality when the breath is front and center. It's amazing how effective one simple tool can be. It can radically change an entire experience. We've just practiced the same exact set of movements and changed only one thing, how we use the breath. The feeling, however, couldn't be more different between the two experiences.

It's only a few words and a reminder to not only breathe generally but about how and when to use your breath effectively to move your body, which takes the pressure off physically, mentally, and emotionally. What a relief!

REFLECTION MOMENT

Now that we've done our first experiment, it's a good time to try being your own guide. You have reflected on the relationship between tension and ease and the breath. We know that we need effort to accomplish something, but when we move with ease, we accomplish more with less effort. We know that we obviously are breathing when we are moving no matter if it's intentional or not, but with the use of the breath as the fuel, we can move easier and accomplish challenges with ease. I encourage you to reflect and take in the concepts we've explored so far.

Feel free to write, move, or explore—whatever works best for you to internalize and experience the breath-body connection. Here are a few questions to get you going:

☆ **When do I feel tension in my life, and what happens to me physically and emotionally when I am tense?**

☆ **Where does tension hang out in my body?**

☆ **When do I feel at ease in my life, and what happens to me physically and emotionally when I am at ease?**

☆ **When do I feel most spacious?**

☆ **What part of my body drops tension first when I begin to relax?**

☆ **Do I feel mostly tense or mostly at ease?**

☆ Would I like to feel more at ease?

☆ Do I find myself using a lot of effort to accomplish tasks and getting frustrated when things don't work out how I planned?

☆ Do I believe a physical practice of moving with ease can shift how I deal with tension in my life?

These are all useful questions to answer only for yourself. This is not a test or a judgment, but simply an opportunity to check in with whatever is happening in your life and how you react in the moment. The more we discover about how we are in the world, the more we are equipped to improve and have a better, more useful experience with our time. This practice is a process and something

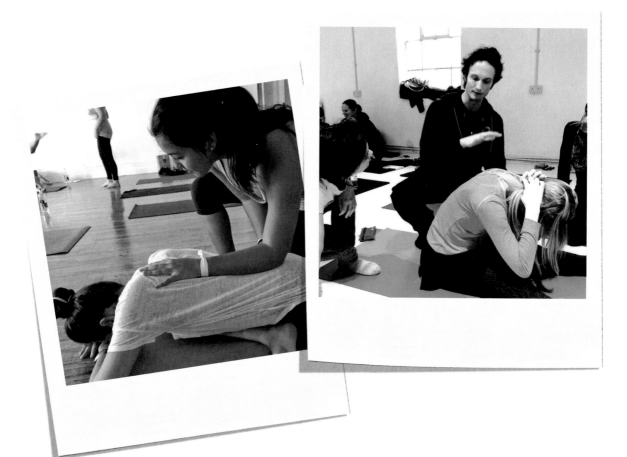

to continue to come back to, check in, and use to connect with yourself. When I come back to these questions and this practice of ease, I immediately become calm, self-aware, and easy, and I slide into the zone of accomplishing more with less effort. Trust me—it's a process, not a destination, and it's important to be kind to yourself during the process. We're all here to improve, help ourselves, and help one another. This is time for you to focus on yourself. Enjoy the space, time, and gift you are giving yourself. Taking this time is the most important practice.

The next time you feel tension creep in—whether it's during your physical practice, when you're at work, having a confrontation with a friend or a co-worker, or an inner dialogue struggle—I encourage you to take a few really full, big, deep breaths. Allow your breath to physically move your body as you inhale and soften as you exhale. This isn't a time-out exercise or a prescription to wait three breaths until you cool down; it's a physical and emotional shift you can easily make anytime you need more space.

You are a space maker; all you need to do is remember how to create that space when you need more of it. You can shift from feeling closed, tight, stuck, and tense to feeling spacious, open, movable, and free with one simple tool in one moment in time. Your breath is a limitless resource that creates more room for you to breathe, feel, and connect with yourself so you can do what you desire in this world. All the tools you need are right inside, waiting for you to discover and use them effectively. We started with the biggest, heaviest-lifting, most multifunction tool we have: the breath. Pretty awesome, isn't it?

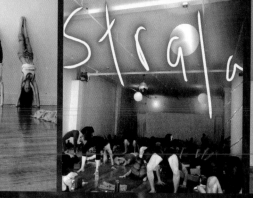
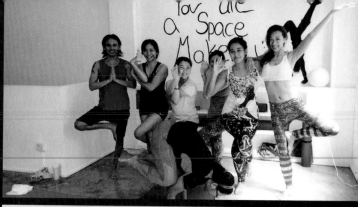
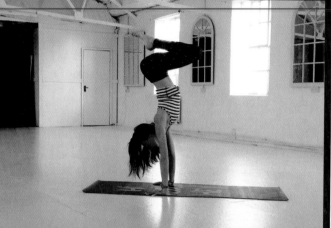
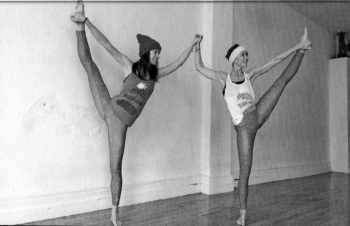
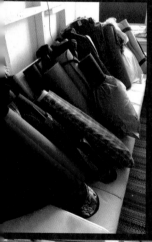
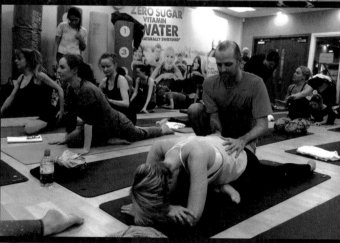
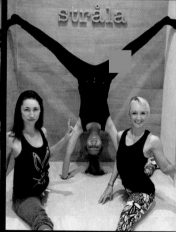
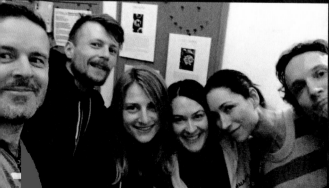
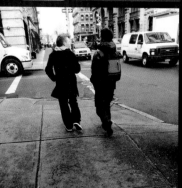
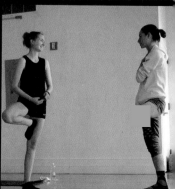

CHAPTER 3

FOLLOW YOUR INTUITION

a reminder to feel

MOVE HOW IT FEELS GREAT TO MOVE.
GET CONNECTED TO YOUR INTUITION.

The next exciting piece in the practice of Strala is the reminder to feel. This empowering concept is all about reminding you to pay attention to what your body is saying so you can respond accordingly. When you pay attention to what you feel and move how it feels great to move, you give yourself the space to relax and heal; your mind has the space to open, calm down, and focus; and you can access greater creativity and inspiration because the stress has just rolled right off. Your entire system can go into restore mode.

Tapping into your intuition on a regular basis is the foundation for healthy self-care, a practice that pays massive dividends both on and off the mat. Paying attention to what your body craves—and it differs day to day—allows you to supply it with the resources it needs to be the best it can be. Sometimes you need to rest. Sometimes you need to move. Sometimes you just need to sit on the couch and watch a movie. If you turn your attention inward, you'll know what will restore and replenish you, making you feel fantastic from the inside out.

Practicing this focus on yourself is essential while moving through the poses when you're in a Strala class. We practice two types of moves: those that happen continuously and those where there is more time and space to linger and settle. In the continuous movements, we focus on moving how it feels great for you. It's not about controlling exactly how you move; it's about helping you experience the movements, which are designed to feel expansive, free, and spacious. There is no beginning or end to them. One shifts to another with no stops and starts in between. In the moves that invite lingering and settling, the aim is to relax and breathe into yourself.

Remember—with the practice of Strala, you are in charge. I remind you to move how it feels great to move, linger where it feels nice to linger, and explore in your body with the goal to find a way that works for you. But you are the boss of you. It's my job to keep you safe and guide you to pay attention to what feels best for you in the moment, but nothing more. I'm just here to help.

CREATING STRUCTURE FOR FREEDOM

A couple of years ago, I was sitting on a big group of rocks by the ocean in Spain pondering the concept of following intuition. This hadn't been my plan. Really I just had an hour in between leading yoga classes at a retreat nearby, so

I decided to sneak out to get some space and quiet my mind. But hey, sometimes deep thoughts happen.

As I sat peacefully on the shore, my attention was drawn to the water as it crashed into the rock formations and gathered in small natural pools. Watching the water, my mind turned to the ideas of structure, boundaries, and freedom. I realized that without the rocks, the water wouldn't be able to gather in these natural pools; it would flow around with the current and the wind. Within the pool the water still moved freely, but it was contained within the structure of the rocks. That's when a cool revelation washed over me like a giant wave. When we provide a safe structure for ourselves, we can experience freedom. When we have no structure, intuition and freedom drift.

If a group of people came into a room, and those people were simply instructed to move how it felt good to move, they would be lost. With no other direction, they'd be wondering what the heck they were supposed to do, and the feeling would be chaos. However, if they were told to move how it felt good to move within a safe, clear structure of certain movements, freedom would be the natural experience. The structure would provide them with the opportunity to look within because they wouldn't have the confusion around what they should be doing.

The Strala concept of a reminder to feel is about giving direction to follow how you feel within the structure of a movement. Just as an animal knows how to shift and flow in the context of running away from a predator, we are able to adjust our movements within the context of going through a routine.

Somewhere along the line we stopped paying attention to our intuition and started to follow strict instructions from others. We stopped listening to how we feel and started doing what we're told, even if it goes against what we think is right.

This blatant disregard to feeling leads to all sorts of problems. When we disconnect from how we feel, we gather tension in our bodies and minds, create a habit of separation from self, and spur on a chain reaction of mental and physical health problems that can engulf our lives.

I'm not interested in telling you how to move or telling you how to feel. What I am interested in is providing a safe and clear structure for you to move how it feels great for you so you can be expansive in your body, mind, and life. Connecting to yourself and allowing your body to do what it needs to do to work out kinks, build strength, and radiate health doesn't come from me telling you where to put your hands or feet.

Health is multifaceted, and part of living a healthy life is giving yourself the space and time to pay attention to how you feel and then leaving room for your body and mind to work for you. This will help you in so many ways—relieving both physical and emotional pain. Moving how it feels great to move will also get you further with less effort because you will be exploring a way that works for your body.

THE SPACE FOR CHOICE

The goal of tapping into your intuition and finding freedom is creating the ability to choose the best path for you. High performers of all kinds—from professional athletes to scientists—talk about a sweet spot of effort that leaves room for creativity. Improvisation and spontaneity are essential for high-level achievement, meaning the "how" of approaching something matters a lot. If we stress out, all our energy is used for stress and worry. But once we choose to listen to our intuition, we lose the stress and we create space for choice. Choice is essential. It's in that space that we can feel into what we need to do to achieve what we desire. It's in that space that we experience the awesome feeling of being "in the zone." Once you choose to follow how you feel, the possibilities are endless.

So the breath-body connection opens up space and room in your body and mind. And then the reminder to feel gives you ideas on exploring in that space with a goal of following your intuition.

In most yoga classes (as well as in life), we have options. In a Strala class we choose which option to take based on what feels great in the moment, instead of what we can or can't do in the moment by pushing ourselves to the limit. It's amazing to watch the difference between a class where I lead an exercise instructing each pose without much choice and a class with loads of freedom to move. Even with the same group of people and the same movements, a whole lot more is accomplished with a lot less effort when feeling is encouraged. Freedom in movement leads to not only feeling great during the process but also seeing more results. You'll get stronger faster by following how you feel. You'll gain more range of motion by staying in positions that feel nice. You'll accomplish challenging poses by exploring instead of following rules.

Here are a few of the reminders I often use to help people feel connection:

☆ **Move how it feels great to move.**

☆ **Follow how you feel.**

☆ **If it feels great, do it. If something else feels better, do that instead.**

☆ **We'll meet up when you're ready.**

All the reminders to feel are designed to spark your creative curiosity and remind you of your freedom to explore, play, and have fun, all while feeling safe within the structure you've created for yourself. We are building something really cool and awesome here. It's an expansive experience from the inside out, and you are front and center.

GETTING PAST THE HICCUPS

So if sensitization and getting into feeling mode are so awesome, why don't we naturally do it? It all goes back to that same mental hurdle we had about ease in general. We've been trained to work hard and suffer through the pain to get the reward. In essence we've been trained to tune out anything our bodies may be telling us. Even if you hear what your body needs, you are told to ignore it. Work as hard as possible, otherwise you won't get what you want. Follow the rules. Fight through. And sometimes it works. Sometimes we fight and get the goal. But often we just get more and more tense and set up stumbling blocks that make that process longer. When we work efficiently with the breath-body connection and incorporate intuition, we change our focus from the goal to the process. The results are blowing past the goal and moving ahead with ease.

If you're finding it hard to get away from the instruction you've gotten throughout your life in order to trust and follow your intuition, just remember that you don't have to do it all at once. Sensitization takes time. Moving according to what you learn when you listen to yourself takes time. There's no three-step plan, no road map, no outline. Starting the process with movement on the mat creates a safe environment for you to explore. Soon enough that exploration will teach you that you are, in fact, the best one to speak for you. You will be able to see what will make you feel good. What will make you healthy. What will make you shine. And in the end, you'll gain more self-confidence and radiate more love.

LET'S PRACTICE!

Now I'm going to take you through a quick routine that will help you see just how tapping into your intuition will change your experience of movement. First I'll take you through the routine using only brief movement phrases. Then I'll take you through the same routine and add reminders to feel. Both routines will incorporate the breath-body connection because that will make the difference even starker. We know how great using the breath to power movement feels, so now we'll see how much better moving can be when you listen to what you need.

WITHOUT REMINDERS TO FEEL

Start in child's pose. Sit your hips to your heels and relax your torso on the ground in front of you. Hang here for a few long, big breaths.

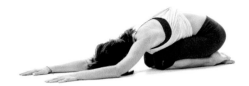

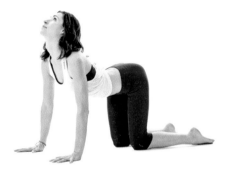 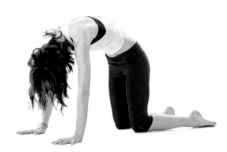

Come onto all fours. Take a big inhale, drop your belly, arch your back, and look upward. Take a long exhale, round your back, and look inward. Move through this a few more times on your own.

Tuck your toes, take a big inhale, and lift your hips up and back to down dog.

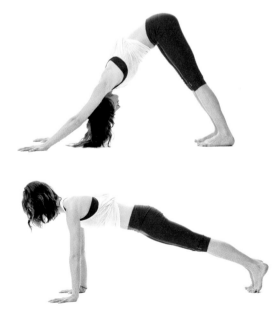

Tuck your chin and roll out to plank pose.

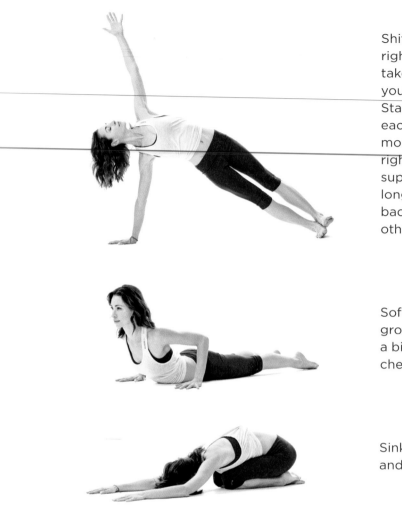

Shift your weight to your right hand, lift your hips up, take a big inhale, and open your body to your left side. Stack your feet on top of each other. If you want some more stability, soften your right shin to the ground for support. Hang here for a few long, deep breaths. Come back to plank and try the other side.

Soften your knees to the ground, sink your hips, take a big inhale, and open your chest forward.

Sink your hips to your heels and relax in child's pose.

How did that feel? Take notice of how you feel mentally and physically. I hope you feel okay and nothing is too wonky. My goal isn't to put you through something that feels awful. I want to show you how a movement that feels normal, and even familiar, changes when you take it to a place of feeling. This first round I took you through specific movements without options. I gave you no room to improvise.

In a class with only movement instructions, doing something different from the instruction given would mean that you are "doing it wrong." Often we get stuck in this mode of right or wrong, and we forget about how we feel. Asking about feeling may seem silly when we put it into practice in something as simple as a side plank, but it means everything when it comes to creating a life that feels fantastic.

Okay, let's try this routine again—this time *with* reminders to feel.

WITH REMINDERS

Start in child's pose. Sit your hips to your heels and relax your torso on the ground in front of you. Sway a bit if that feels good to you. Hang here for a few long, big breaths.

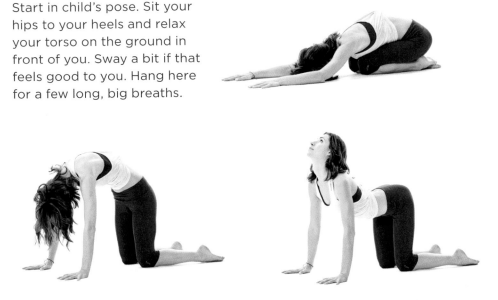

Staying easy in your body, when you're ready, bring yourself onto all fours.
Roll around your torso how it feels good for you, arching and rounding your spine with your breath. Linger where it feels nice.
Move with this for a few long, deep breaths.

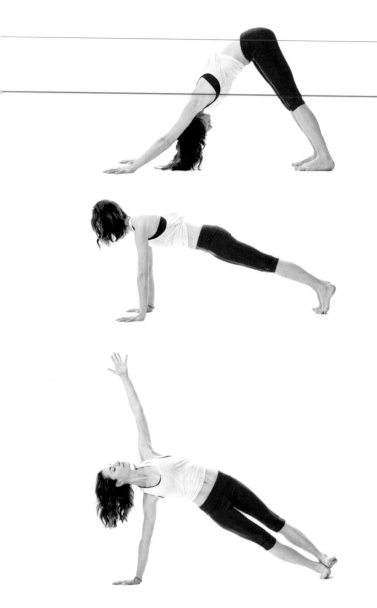

When you're ready, tuck your toes, take a big inhale, and lift your hips up and back to down dog.

Tuck your chin and roll out to your plank pose. Sway a bit side to side or forward and back if that feels nice.

Shift your weight to your right hand, lift your hips up, take a big inhale, and open your body to your left side. Maybe stay here or lift the top leg up or lower your bottom shin down, however feels nice for you. If you want some more stability, soften your right shin to the ground for support. Hang here for a few long, deep breaths. Come back to plank and try the other side.

When you're ready, tuck your chin and roll out into plank. Soften your knees to the ground; sink your hips toward the ground. Maybe look over one shoulder and then the other to open up a bit. If this doesn't feel nice on your lower back, soften your elbows even more, opening up your middle and upper back. Take a big inhale and open your chest forward.

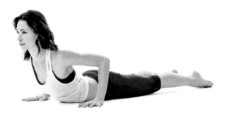

Soften your hips to your heels and relax in child's pose. Let everything rest here for a few moments.

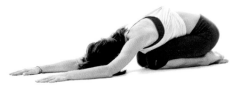

How did that feel? Hopefully you felt a nice sense of freedom to move how it felt good to you. Hopefully you didn't feel as if you had to stick to any pose that wasn't useful or didn't feel good.

This idea of moving how it feels good is an interesting and ever-unfolding concept. One layer is about backing off from something that doesn't feel good and moving farther into something that does feel good. This practice allows the body's kinks to be worked out naturally and strength to be built easily. Another layer is about ignoring physical goals and resting in feeling mode. And yet another layer is about getting really involved in the process rather than simply going through the motions.

Reminders to feel aren't orders or instructions to do a certain thing at a certain time. The magic in using reminders instead of instructions is their power of suggestion to ignite your own feeling, opening up all that room for improvisation.

The reminders are designed to help connect you to yourself, get you in the habit of self-care, and cultivate creativity and exploration when you are approaching simple and challenging movements alike. They are designed to put you completely in charge of how, when, and what you are doing with your body.

You may have noticed in the second routine that time went by a lot faster—even if the routine actually took longer to do. Cues such as "when you are ready" are meant to give you the time you need to move into the pose. The phrase is designed with space so you can explore. Without the reminders any space that exists is filled with holding the pose and waiting to do the next one. The reminders help suspend the concept of time to shift you into feeling and exploring. When you spend time feeling and moving how it feels great to move instead of staying in a pose and waiting until the next one comes along, time goes by incredibly fast, and the challenges during the movements become lighter, easier, and more freeing.

Feeling has a lot to do with when and how. The timing of when something feels right for us makes a huge difference in all aspects of our lives. Sometimes it's appropriate to keep things moving, and sometimes it's better to linger. When all your attention is placed on feeling, you're going to get some pretty spectacular results on your mat and in your life.

AND NOW FOR A CHALLENGE

If you enjoyed that exercise, here is a routine that is designed to help you see even more how feeling can change how you experience movement. Again we'll do two versions of the same routine: one without reminders and one with them. If you're a beginner, there are some moves in here that are going to be beyond your reach. Let's face it, a handstand isn't something everyone can do. But try this out. Do what you can do, and see how it feels to move through the challenges while in feeling mode. Just remember: stay easy in your body and mind. Feel free to rest when you need to and come back to the routine when you are ready.

WITHOUT REMINDERS TO FEEL

Start in child's pose. Sit your hips to your heels and relax your torso on the ground in front of you. Hang here for a few long, big breaths.

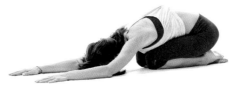

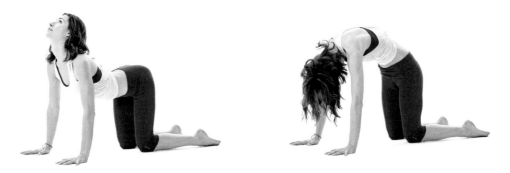

Come onto all fours. Take a big inhale, drop your belly, arch your back, and look upward. Take a long exhale, round your back, and look inward. Move through this a few more times on your own.

Tuck your toes, take a big inhale, and lift your hips up and back to down dog.

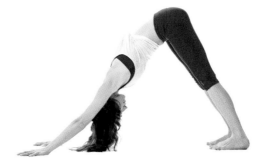

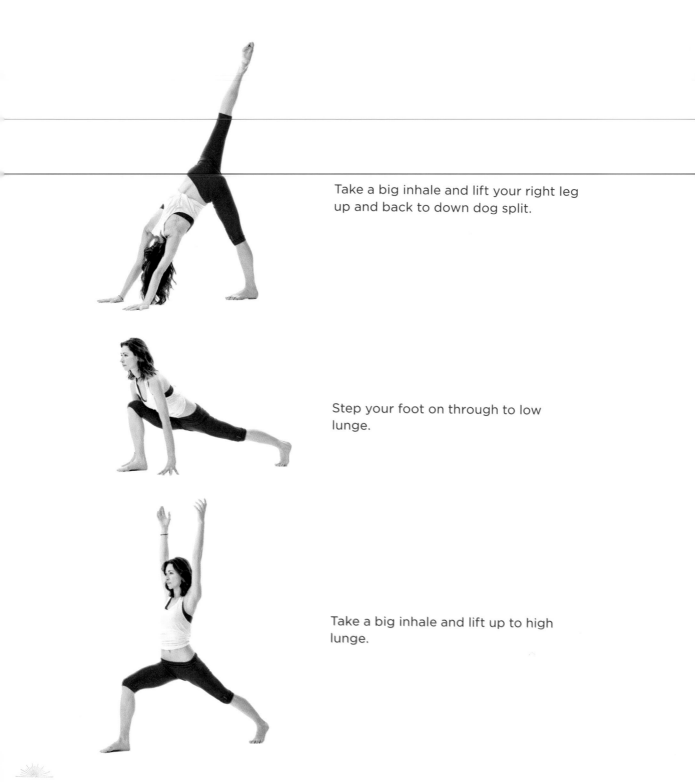

Take a big inhale and lift your right leg up and back to down dog split.

Step your foot on through to low lunge.

Take a big inhale and lift up to high lunge.

Exhale and twist toward your front leg and open your arms wide out to your sides.

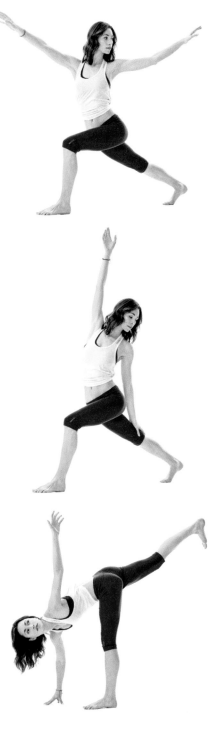

Tip back and reverse the twist, sliding your back hand down your back leg and extending your top arm up.

Lean forward and tip into twisted half-moon, bringing your fingertips to the ground. Extend your back leg long behind you. Open your top arm up and gaze upward.

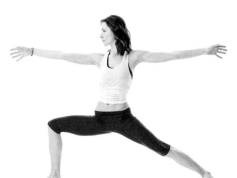

Press your right fingertips into the ground and open your body to your left. Open your left arm up and roll your body open.

Step your top foot back to warrior 2. Turn your back toes in toward your front toes. Sink your hips low so your front knee bends over your front toes. Extend your arms out to your sides. Hang here for a few long, deep breaths.

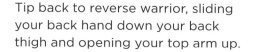

Tip back to reverse warrior, sliding your back hand down your back thigh and opening your top arm up.

Tip your torso forward and press your right forearm on your right thigh. Spin your torso upward. Extend your left arm up and overhead. Gaze upward toward your top hand.

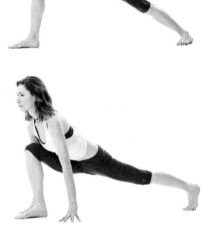

Press your fingertips on the ground on either side of your front foot. Sink your hips low.

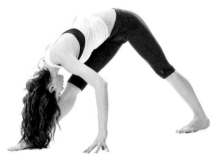

Keeping your fingertips on the ground, lift your hips up and relax your torso over your front leg.

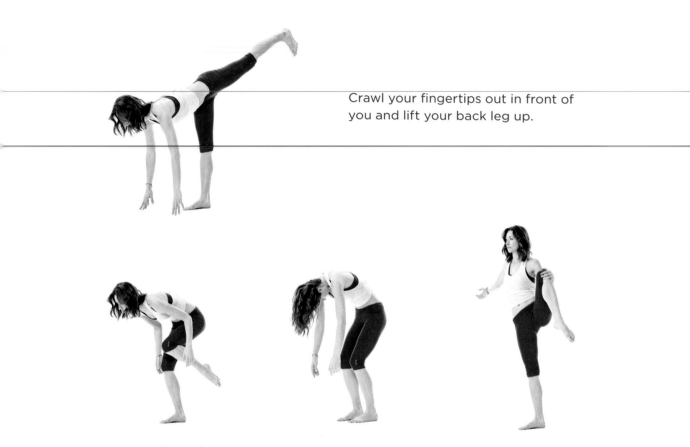

Crawl your fingertips out in front of you and lift your back leg up.

Round up to stand and hug your left shin into your chest.
Take a big inhale and give your shin a squeeze.

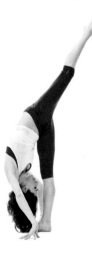

Take a dive over your front leg, pressing your fingertips into the ground for your standing split. Relax your head and neck.

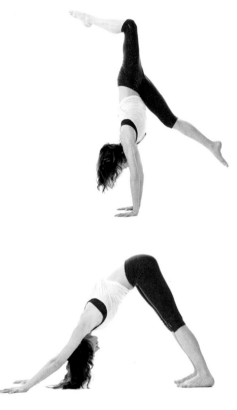

Plant your palms on the ground about a foot or so in front of your front foot. Rock forward and back, getting your hips over your shoulders. Rock back and forth a few times.

Come back to down dog.

Repeat on the other side.

Okay, how did that feel? Hopefully not too awful because at least we were moving along fueled with the breath. Did you notice any freedom missing, or did you feel okay in the movements?

Honestly, when I lead workshops, it pains me to lead this version. I feel as if I am in a position of senseless authority, telling people what to do and where to go, giving no option for a softer way, without a good reason why. Of course structure needs to exist for the experience to feel safe, but as you'll experience with our next version, adding the reminders to feel creates a much nicer and more open sequence.

Before you head to the next routine, take a moment to reflect on how this first one felt to you. Write about it in your journal if you'd like a reminder in the future.

When you're ready, move on to the routine with the reminders to feel, and see if you feel any difference.

WITH REMINDERS TO FEEL

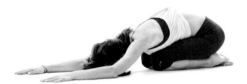

Start in child's pose. Sit your hips to your heels and relax your torso on the ground in front of you. Sway a little side to side if that feels good for you. Hang here for a few long, big breaths.

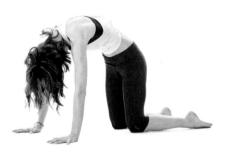

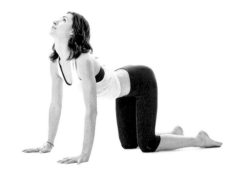

When you're ready, come onto all fours, moving easy on your joints and on the rest of you. Take a few soft movements in your spine here, maybe side to side, or round and round, or forward and back, breathing really big and full and deep. Move how it feels good to move in your spine.

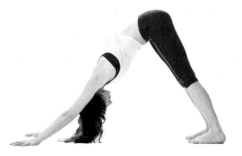

When you're ready, tuck your toes, take a big inhale, and lift your hips up and back to down dog.

Take a big inhale and lift your
right leg up and back to down
dog split. Open up your hips and
shoulders if that feels good.

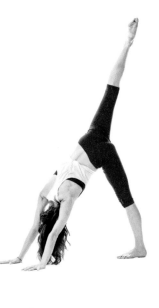

Step your foot on through to
low lunge.

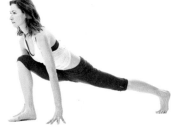

Take a big inhale and lift up
to high lunge.

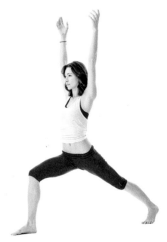

Exhale and twist to your front leg and open your arms wide out to your sides.

Tip back and reverse the twist, sliding your back hand down your back leg and extending your top arm up.

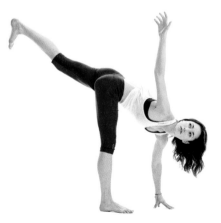

Lean forward and tip into your twisted half-moon, bringing your left fingertips to the ground. Open up toward your right side. Gaze upward if that feels nice.

Press your right fingertips into the ground and open your body to your left. Open your left arm up and roll your body open.

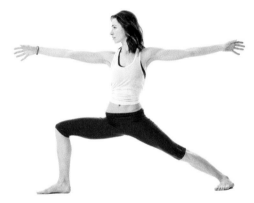

Step your top foot back to your warrior 2. Turn your back toes in toward your front toes. Sink your hips low so your front knee bends over your front toes. Extend your arms out to your sides. Hang here for a few long, deep breaths, swaying around a bit if that feels nice.

Tip back to your reverse warrior, sliding your back hand down your back thigh and opening your top arm up.

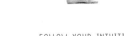

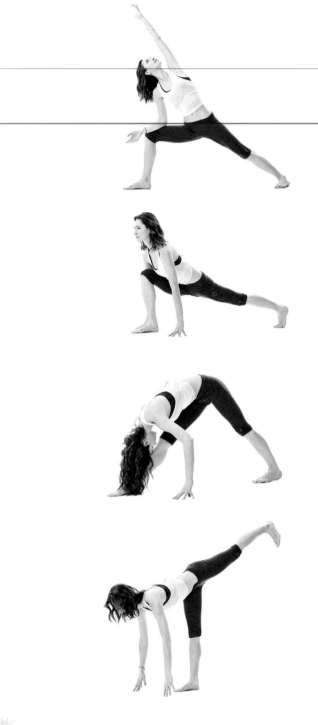

Tip your torso forward and press your right forearm on your right thigh. Spin your torso upward. Extend your left arm up and overhead.

Press your fingertips on the ground on either side of your front foot. Sink your hips low. Sway a little side to side if that feels good.

Keeping your fingertips on the ground, lift your hips up and relax your torso over your front leg.

Crawl your fingertips out in front of you and float your back leg up.

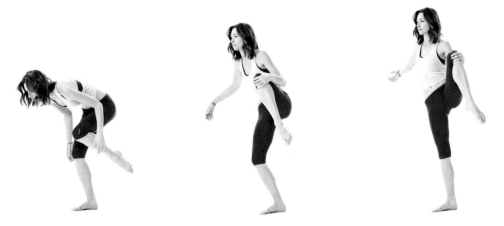

Round up to stand and hug your left shin into your chest.
Take a big inhale and give your shin a squeeze.
Roll around in your hips if that feels nice.

Take a dive over your front leg,
pressing your fingertips into the
ground for your standing split.
Relax your head and neck. Sway
a little here.

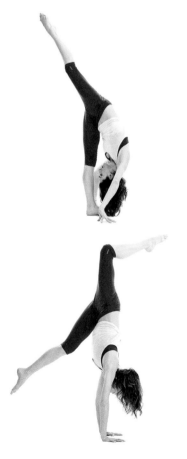

Plant your palms on the ground
about a foot or so in front of
your front foot. Rock forward
and back, getting your hips over
your shoulders. Rock back and
forth a few times here, rolling
around in your hips and belly.

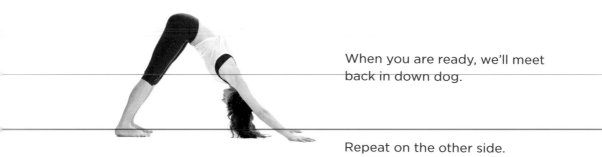

When you are ready, we'll meet back in down dog.

Repeat on the other side.

All right, now how did *that* feel? Was the experience different? Hopefully you felt more encouraged to explore the second go-around. Remember, feeling gets you more than posing. If you allow yourself to feel the movements instead of putting your body in the shapes, you'll get further faster, and the process is so much more fun.

The goal of the Strala classes is to connect you back to yourself. The movements are designed to build a strong, mobile body and a calm, focused mind. The class is set up for you to enjoy the entire experience. Of course, certain movements will be challenging, but what makes the challenge enjoyable is the way you are guided to approach it. Supported by the breath and reminded to explore, challenges become easy to accomplish.

REFLECTION MOMENT

Now that we're simmering in feeling mode, it's a nice time to take this a step further and consider how all this sensitization applies to life. You have experienced the difference that a practice of feeling makes in a yoga routine. When we give ourselves the space and time to move how it feels good, we open up endless possibilities. I encourage you to take a moment to reflect and take in the concepts we have explored so far.

Feel free to move a bit more on your own to internalize the experience. If writing down your thoughts calls to you, grab your journal and write how you feel. Here are a few questions to get you going:

- ☆ Are there times and situations where I feel disconnected from feeling?

- ☆ What happens to me physically and mentally when I feel disconnected?

- ☆ When do I feel the most connected in my life?

- ☆ What happens to me physically and mentally when I feel connected?

- ☆ When do I feel most free?

- ☆ What part of my body feels the most freedom?

- ☆ In my regular life, do I follow my intuition most of the time, or do I follow the rules?

- ☆ Would I like to feel more connected to my intuition?

- ☆ Do I often feel rushed or late? Do I have a negative connection with time?

- ☆ Do I believe a physical practice of following how I feel can shift how I deal with navigating my life?

In my view, following your intuition is one of the most powerful things you can do to put your life on its best path. You need to move in a way that is good for you. Reminders to feel during classes help you do this on the mat. They celebrate individuality within the safety of a structure. And they have the awesome result of connecting you to how you feel during your whole practice, which keeps you connected in your life. It's not too tough to imagine a life where you have room to breathe and move freely. The space and awesome vibes that are created by listening to your intuition help you with clear decision making, authentic connections to those around you, and living in alignment with your passion. When you feel disconnected from yourself, you can come back to the practice of moving how it feels good to move on the mat. You'll soften right back to your most in-touch, sensitized self in no time. Remember to start with a big, deep inhale to create space and a long, easy exhale to move in.

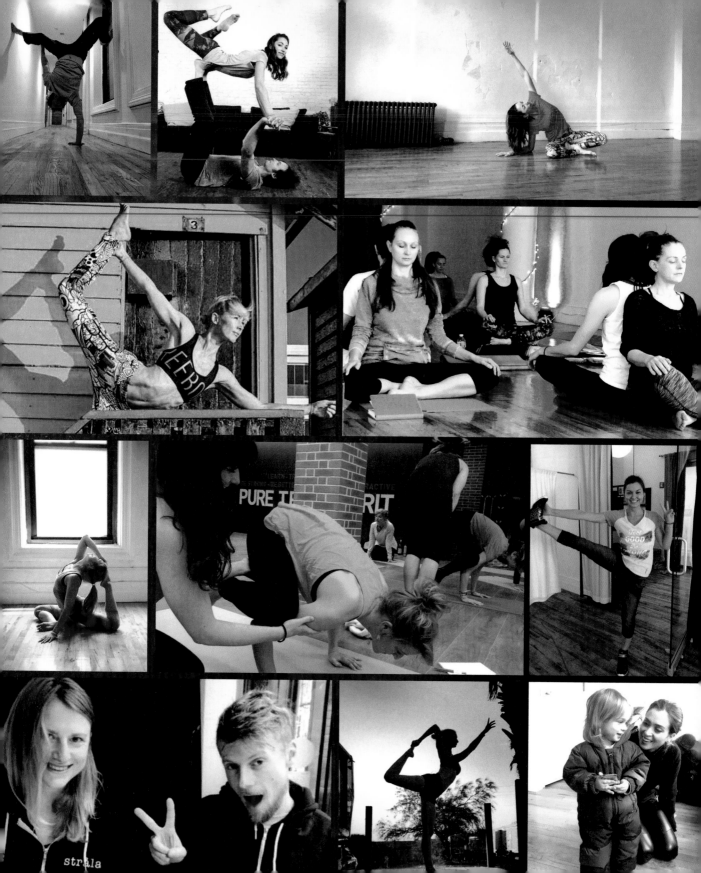

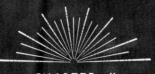

CHAPTER 4

GET IN THE FLOW

finding natural movement

MOVING FROM THE MIDDLE—
ENJOYING A POWERFUL INTERNAL EXPERIENCE.

HOPEFULLY you're experiencing how the first two elements of Strala blend together to deliver an enjoyable, easygoing process. Our final element is the grand concept of natural movement. The principles of natural movement will entertain a lifetime of growth and possibilities.

Natural movement, as opposed to technique-based steps needed to achieve a pose, embodies an overall approach of moving easily, with everything you've got, in every direction you can, starting from your center. When we apply step-by-step techniques to achieve a position—such as rotate your thigh, flex your feet, engage your arms, and kick your leg—we practice immobilizing our entire self, both body and mind, which means that we can't accomplish much of anything. At best we might stick a pose, after senselessly putting ourselves in a narrow hallway of possibility and a lot of fussing around. The pose, and only one expression of it, eclipses all else when these techniques are applied. We settle on the external position as the goal, which detracts from the value of practicing yoga. However, by practicing natural movement, the process of achieving not only the pose but also every possibility around and beyond it becomes your reality. We all want more with less effort, and natural movement is the approach that takes us there.

With natural movement, we soften as we move, moving initially from the hips and belly. The rest of the body follows. Movement becomes slow, soft, and continuous. This waterlike approach will take you to a place of heightened body awareness and an improved sense of space, body, and position, and it will allow you to do this more easily. Take away natural movement, and we're simply trying to put our bodies into poses in any way we can, flailing around, sweating, and out of control. External movements are frazzled, fear based, and stressed.

Natural movement is about working from the middle, moving every way possible through the structure of the motion, and expanding your circle of comfort. You improve gradually yet swiftly. There is no working outside your comfort zone. There is no "close your eyes and just go for the pose." There is no "just wait it out until it's over." You're sensitizing yourself to each and every piece of your movement. You're sustainably expanding your sphere of what's possible through committing to the process instead of forcing a pose. It's ninja stuff, really. This grace is what gives off the impression that what you're doing is simple. Natural movement is the key to having a powerful internal experience, and in many ways it's the most critical ingredient to the process.

NATURAL MOVEMENT

While breathing and paying attention to the sensations in your body help you feel better while moving, the focus of this piece of the Strala philosophy is the movement itself. It is the approach we take toward movement—the how of the movement. And this approach is based in concepts in nature.

As I already noted, natural movement is all about softening. But it's also about support and flow. What do I mean by this? Think about how nature moves. A tree doesn't tense itself to resist the wind; it remains soft and flexible yet supported, so it can bend and sway in the breeze. Water doesn't force itself to go in a straight line; it winds its way through rocks and valleys, moving in whichever direction is easiest.

The approach of natural movement focuses on softening our joints and muscles as we move and initiating movement from the middle of our bodies, our hips and bellies, so we remain fully supported. Natural movement guides us to move efficiently with the least amount of effort. It also helps us move through each moment with ease, making the whole process of moving more enjoyable.

The other element in how we move—circular rather than linear movement—means that in Strala, we don't aim at poses as end points. The poses are there, but they are no more important than every other inch that we move through. So we move without pose goals. We're not trying to get anywhere; we're already here! In this way, Strala brings us directly into the present, rather than trying to be somewhere else. The movement is completely fluid, both within each pose and from one to the next. There is no end point to a pose, only a shift to the next pose. Just like a tree doesn't blow left, stop, and then blow right, we do not pose, hold, and then move to another pose. In Strala we do *movement phrases*—a term I evolved from the dance world. These phrases take you on a journey of movement with the start and end points being attached to a set of movements rather than a single pose. These movement phrases inspire you to move like a tree, swaying with the breeze and moving from the inside out.

Understanding a bit more about what's involved in natural movement—along with some principles that inspire it—will help you take things to the next level. It will make your life, your movement, and your headspace flow a lot better.

UNNATURAL MOVEMENT

Before we dive even more deeply into natural movement, let's take a look at its opposite: unnatural movement. This happens when we move from the outside in; we lead with our limbs, focus on our extremities, and by doing this we lose the ability to move easily and efficiently. Movement becomes a performance or a flourish, which is great for a balletic line, but for our nonperformance, internal, world-enriching, and self-improvement purposes, natural movement rules.

Unnatural movement often happens because we think we need to flex and engage our muscles to get the most out of a movement or even to perform it correctly. A "need to flex to achieve" mind-set turned into physicality puts tension in the body and mind. It places us in a box and dramatically prohibits movement. When we flex our bodies, we are technically restricting movement. We are unable to move to our full capacity. This not only keeps us more distant from our goals but also adds emotional tension that will in turn show up in our movements. When we move unnaturally, whatever we are doing becomes about suffering through.

Additionally, flexing and engaging kill your ability to improvise to find ease. It puts us in a narrow path of being able to achieve a pose only through a step-by-step process like the following:

1. Flex your abs.

2. Engage your thigh.

3. Kick up.

4. Flex your toes.

5. Jump.

When you put yourself in a tight process, there is only one way to do something, which is likely not a natural way for you. That means the ability to move naturally goes away.

I'm not sure why the idea that we have to flex and tighten our bodies in order to get the most out of our movements has become so prevalent. I'm guessing it has to do with the same fight-to-succeed idea we discussed before. And, yes, there are times when flexing and engaging are good—if you're a linebacker defending a row of intruders in a football game, forming that barrier with your muscles is incredibly useful. But if you are moving through a yoga class with the goal of building strength, creating a healthy range of motion, and reducing stress, natural movement becomes your best friend.

A MIND-BODY CONNECTION

I want to talk here about the connection between the mind and movement. We saw how the flex-and-engage idea hurt our quest for ease. This is because how we think and feel emotionally translates into how we move physically and how we experience our lives. Flex and engage is based in tension, and so when we move with this idea in mind, we move tensely. If we can move to a concept of ease in our minds, we will get ease in our movements. In other words, how we are in our internal worlds can be seen clearly in how we are in our bodies.

Most of us have something we have to overcome to get to the sweet spot of moving naturally. That something is unique for each of us, and working through it is a huge learning experience. Personally my block has been (and, if I'm not careful, continues to be) insecurity and the need to prove my value to myself. It's a tricky quality that I've been able to manage through careful observation and practice. Now most of the time it's just a supporting actor in my performance rather than the star.

Back when I lived with constant insecurity, I moved more comfortably from the outside in. My need to show myself and others that I was worthy was a "neck sticking out" posture, which translated into similar movements and reactions. My limbs would move first. I would be the first one to jump up and grab something in a fast and almost jerky way. Grace and body awareness got left on the back burner and covered up by the need for me to pull myself in all directions. When I addressed my insecurity and worked to embody natural movement, I found my center.

One amazing result of regularly practicing natural movement is the ability to transform our internal challenges into mindful observations. If we can see our weaknesses, we can use them to bring our lives back to balance. From the years of work I've done, I can now identify when my insecurity is about to bubble up.

So, as you can see, moving naturally isn't about just getting strong, healthy, and radiant—though these things do come through natural movement. It is about balancing how we are in our internal worlds; shifting the conversations we have with ourselves to be kind, open, and thoughtful; and broadening our possibilities by unblocking our lives. We are designed to move naturally with the ability to move unnaturally if we choose. It's crucial to our growth that we compassionately observe our minds and our movements so we can evolve into the best versions of ourselves.

AN INTERNAL EXPERIENCE

For purposes of self-reflection and exploration, it's important to have an internal experience when we practice. We want to have the focus go to how we are feeling, what we are doing, and the motivation behind our moves. Moving naturally opens the space for an internal experience. It plays with our ability to tap into intuition to figure out what we truly need.

A shift to sensitization of how we feel and a desire to feel great internally ring clear when time is spent exploring an internal practice. Self-care naturally shifts into priority. Time for cooking and preparing healthy foods, reflection, and meditation naturally become a desire and priority. We experience a shift from attachment to physical things to an excitement for feelings of ease, calm, and space. And this shift helps us drop a lot of the baggage we can accumulate in a lifetime. Natural movement is a tool to help you make a shift in your mind that will then help you move more naturally. Again . . . we have a good circle.

What do natural movements look like? They are designed to bring you back inside so you can connect with yourself. There is no need to flex muscles to feel the burn or achieve a pose. Your body will work for you, your muscles will activate, and you don't need to do anything to make that happen. Doing something to make it happen (flexing and tightening from the outside in) brings attention to the external and goes right to our thoughts. Am I strong enough, flexing enough, doing this right? Flexing creates armor around us and inhibits movement.

Natural movements involve softening into the move and initiating the move from your center. These concepts will carry you to and from any pose you desire. There is no need for stress or tension when it comes to cultivating an internal experience. In fact, stress and tension draw you into the external world. If you place your attention on the outside edges of your body, it brings you out of your internal experience, both physically and emotionally, and inhibits your body from moving with ease. For our purposes, yoga is not a performance or a show of strength, flexibility, or contortion. It is a simple flowing movement where challenging poses and transitions are approached with ease.

A SIMPLE EXPERIMENT

Let's put this concept of having an internal experience into practice without getting too much into the yogalike movements just yet. This is a simple experiment that is designed to get us moving naturally and comfortably without worrying about achieving a pose. The process is focused on exploration and ease. Get ready to drop right into feeling mode and enjoy!

Stand up tall with your feet a bit apart.

Get comfortable. Soften your knees.

Relax your head and neck and shoulders. Relax your arms and hips.

Move from your hips and belly a bit to settle your whole self in.

Roll around your shoulders and let your arms move easy for a bit.

Let everything be loose and easy.

Let your movements settle and soften into stillness for a moment.

Close your eyes and draw your attention inward.

Soften your knees and relax your head, neck, and shoulders.

Take a big inhale and float your arms up overhead.

Press your palms together and bring your thumbs to your heartbeat.

Let yourself soften here for a moment.

If it feels good, let your body shift and drift a little side to side
and easy forward and back.

When you are ready, gently open your eyes and
relax your arms by your sides.

How did that feel? I hope you felt easy in your body, fluid, natural, calm, and relaxed. When you move naturally, you embody fluidity, moving like water, flowing freely, easily, and softly.

❋

FROM HERE TO HERE

Transitions—from one pose to another—are an important focus of natural movement. Unnatural movement often starts and stops. It is this pose, and then this pose, and then this pose—all separate things without any attention paid to how you get from one to the next. But with natural movement, it's a flow. Everything is connected, and finding the path of ease during transition from one pose to the next is loads of fun.

Transitions are great places for exploration because they are ever present. In movement—and in life for that matter—we are in constant transition, shifting from one place to another. Focusing on transitions means focusing on the process and on the present moment. Perhaps in the process of moving from one pose to the next you feel a place where it would be good to linger. You can do that because transitions aren't simply the means to an end; they are wonderful things all on their own. There are, in fact, no moments in between because each moment is a destination, and none of them are final. When we pay attention to exactly where we are in the moment, things get really great. You learn to do just what you need in order to feel your best. Even when you are settling into a resting pose, you breathe and soften into stillness. There is movement even in stillness. As long as we are alive and breathing, we are constantly moving.

When we forget about natural movement, we start to feel stuck. Things require more energy to accomplish, which leaves us more worn-out than we need to be. When we move the most naturally, we get the most out of the experience. Our movements become smooth and oceanic instead of linear and clunky. They simply become easier. When we employ the process of softening as we move, balance comes. The experience becomes circular and uplifting instead of point A to point B, start to finish. The emotional result is improved calmness, creativity, freedom, and focus of mind.

The key in practicing natural movement is to cultivate the flow so it can be most useful and enjoyable to us in our bodies, minds, and lives. On a practical level, this starts with softening before and during a movement. Softening our knees, hips, and joints as we step from place to place. Rolling in our hips and belly as we round from place to place. Always breathing, lifting, softening, one into the next with effortless ease. Movement flows like water. It's continuous, easy, and circular. If you've ever watched a group of tai chi practitioners move in unison, you've seen circular movement. It's relaxing and uplifting to watch. There is no beginning and no end, just constant flow. When you practice natural movement, you become so sensitized to the movements you are making that you can actually feel the air around you as you lift and soften your body. You can move more easily and you have more choice in direction when you start from a soft place. In Strala, we apply the concept of natural movement by softening everything before we move.

Here are a few ways to visualize the natural movement experience:

☆ **Soften as you move.**

☆ **Moving from your hips and belly.**

☆ **Roll around a bit as you move.**

☆ **There is always movement in balance.**

OTHER BENEFITS OF NATURAL MOVEMENT

Natural movement does more than simply help us have an internal experience to create balance in our minds and our lives. It also prevents injuries because natural movements are safe movements. The breath-body connection plus intuition plus natural movement is a formula for a safe experience of expansive awesomeness.

When it comes to safety, joints and big muscle groups come to mind. Wrists, knees, and ankles can take quite a beating when we abandon natural movement. When we move naturally, it becomes second nature to move in ways that are healing. When we move externally or unnaturally, we leave ourselves open for injury. Practicing while frustrated with where we are and wanting change to happen instantly brings jerky, frustrated movements. When we force our bodies to make a certain shape to achieve a yoga pose, we take ourselves out of natural movement and risk pulling and tearing our bodies. This affects us both physically and mentally.

Another cool aspect of natural movement is similar to what we discussed in Chapter 3: it helps us focus on the process instead of the goal, which gives us more results with less effort, not to mention an enjoyable experience.

LET'S PRACTICE!

I think you get the idea about what natural movement is, and I bet you want to get started doing some. Here are some simple movements you can get right into to practice moving naturally. I'm not going to take you through two versions of this exercise, like I did in Chapters 2 and 3. Hopefully you're still feeling soft and fluid from our simple experiment. There is no need to swim upstream. All right . . . take a deep breath and enjoy the ride!

Stand with your feet wide apart. Turn your right toes out and left toes slightly in. Take a big inhale and open your arms out to your sides. Exhale and soften your hips and settle into warrior 2. Hang here for a few long, deep breaths. Soften your back knee, relax your arms down by your sides, and roll around in your hips and belly a bit to turn this into an easygoing hip opener. When you find a nice, comfortable warrior 2, take a big inhale and open your arms back out to your sides.

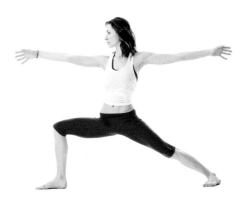

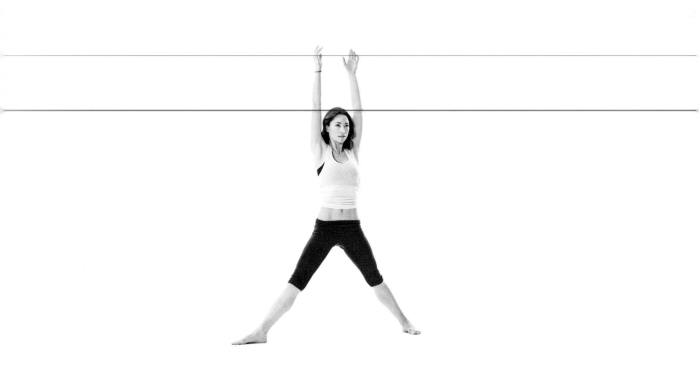

Take a big inhale and lift your hips and arms up. Exhale and soften back into warrior 2, softening both knees as you settle back in. Let your arms relax down by your sides and be easy. Take a few moments here to move around and be easy. Roll around your shoulders and head and neck to find a nice, comfortable place. Try this out a few more times, inhaling, lifting up, and softening back in.

Now find warrior 2 in the easiest way possible. Find a way of being strong and soft simultaneously. There is a fine balance of effort where if you let just an ounce of it go, you wouldn't be in the movement anymore and if you added just a tad, you would have more effort than you need. Make it a quest to find that balance. When we find the easiest way to accomplish movements, we find harmony in our bodies and minds, and we are able to find the easiest ways to accomplish all kinds of things in our lives. This is where our fun transformations happen with ease!

MOVING WITH THE ELEMENTS

Now that you've experienced the simple transition between warrior 2 and warrior 2 lift, I want to guide you through a bit longer—yet still easy—routine so you can experience transitions even more.

In this routine I'll use quite a few reminders to feel, and I'll incorporate breathing instructions. These will help bring your attention to how you can access natural movement. You'll be reminded that your inhale fuels the movement and lifts you up. Your exhale softens and moves you further along. You are reminded to move how it feels good within each moment and pay attention to how you feel so you can fully enjoy yourself. You'll also turn on the relaxation response and reset your entire system, gaining loads of positive energy while you practice.

When we move naturally from the middle, rolling around in our hips and bellies, we embody fluidity and can accomplish anything with ease.

Stand up nice and tall. Soften your knees. Relax your head and neck and shoulders. Bring your palms together and press your thumbs to your heartbeat. Close your eyes for a moment and settle in here. Allow yourself to shift and drift a little side to side or easy forward and back, moving how it feels nice. Soften here for a few more moments.

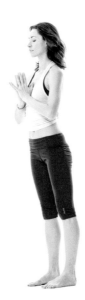

When you're ready, take a big inhale, lifting up a bit; exhale and soften a little easier. Take a big inhale and lift your arms up overhead. Exhale and relax your arms by your sides. Soften your knees as you move.

Shift your weight onto your right leg, take a big inhale, and hug your left shin into your chest. Roll around in your hips and belly, moving your hugged shin around how it feels good to you.

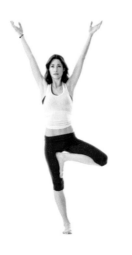

Press the bottom of your foot either into your upper thigh, or onto your calf so your toes are resting on the ground. However is most comfortable for you. Take a big inhale and lift your arms up. Allow your body to shift and drift in the breeze how it feels good for you.

When you're ready, hug your shin back into your chest, rolling your leg around how it feels good to you.

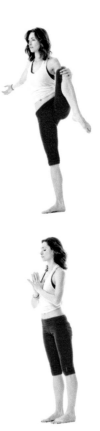

When you're ready, place your foot back down and come to standing. Bring your palms together and your thumbs to your heartbeat. Soften your knees, head, neck, and shoulders. Close your eyes and move a bit here softly if it feels good. When you're ready, open your eyes.

How was that for you? Were you able to stay in the moment and move how it felt great to move? It's amazing that even in a simple routine natural movement makes all the difference. It keeps you focused on the process instead of the goal and keeps your mind and body from packing on tension.

A LITTLE MORE OF A CHALLENGE

Okay! Let's try something a bit tougher. The same ideas apply to this routine: stay present, explore transitions to find a path of ease, and move how it feels good to move. Make sure to soften while you move and make transition moments feel enjoyable rather than clunky and harsh. These in-between moments are my personal favorites. When we enjoy the in-between times just as much as the main event, the practice—and life—gets really fun.

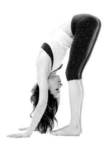

Come into an easy standing forward bend with soft knees. Relax your torso over your legs. Let your head and neck relax and your arms drape down easy. Sway your torso a bit side to side and move how it feels good to you to move. If you find a place that is holding a bit of tension, linger there for a moment. Breathe big and full and deep. Hang here for a few long, deep breaths to open things up.

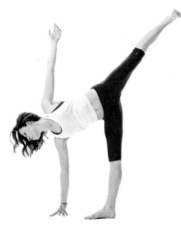

Soften your knees, press your right fingertips to the ground, take a big inhale, and open from your middle, opening your hips and torso toward your left and extending your left leg behind you and your left arm up to half-moon. Exhale and return to standing forward bend. Roll through this a few times to get the feeling of the natural movement.

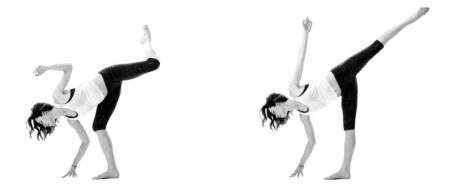

From half-moon, exhale and soften your knees and your elbows and relax right here in the movement. Like a balloon that lets out a little air, let everything soften and relax. Inhale and open back to half-moon, extending outward through the middle of your body on outward through your feet and fingertips. Roll through this a few times to get the feel of softening and opening.

From half-moon, soften your knees, elbows, and everything a bit. Slide your top leg back until your foot reaches the ground a few feet behind you; angle your back toes slightly in. Press down through your legs and take a big inhale to lift your torso up.

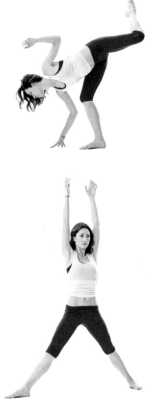

Press down through your legs, take a big inhale, and lift your hips, torso, and arms up.

Exhale and soften into warrior 2. Open your arms out to your sides, gazing gently over your front fingers. Sink your hips low, bending your front knee so it stacks on top of your front ankle. Extend your back leg strong, angling your back toes in slightly.

Take a big inhale and tip your torso back toward your back leg. Slide your back hand gently down your back leg for stability. Extend your opposite arm up. Allow your hips to lift naturally as you lean back.

As you exhale sweep your torso forward toward your front foot; soften your knees as you shift your body forward. Crawl your fingertips out in front of you until your left foot starts to lift off the ground. When you feel balanced, take a big inhale and open everything up and out, extending your left arm up and your left leg back. Play around a few times with opening and closing your extended arm and leg into your torso with your breath. Keep your knees soft as you move. Let your whole body be easy and movable. Don't worry about what the pose looks like; simply enjoy the movement, and let your body naturally find the place where it feels good to linger.

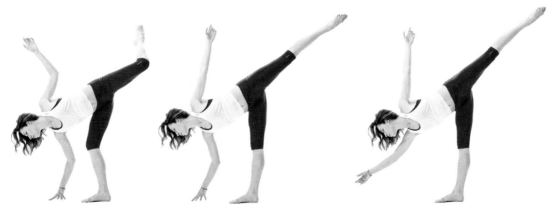

Pressing your right fingertips on the ground, extend your back
leg behind you and your lifted arm up, opening your torso to your side.
Gaze up toward your top hand if that feels good. If looking up doesn't
feel great, gaze down or straight out to your side.

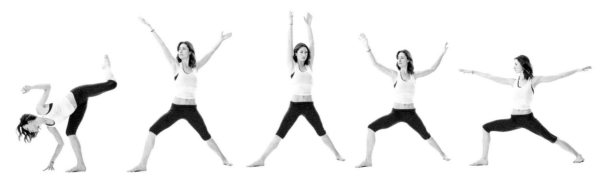

Now we'll bring it back to warrior 2. Soften both knees and reach
your top leg toward the ground so much that your fingertips start to lift off
the ground. Once your foot reaches the ground, press down through your
legs and take a big inhale to lift everything up. Inhale and lift your hips
and arms up. Exhale and soften back to warrior 2.

Move through this transition a few times with your own breath and enjoy
the softness of your movements. When you find ways of moving from one foot
to the other, from one hand to the other, or foot to hand, hand to foot with ease,
you can do pretty much anything with ease. Getting the movements easier in

your body isn't so much about gaining strength as it is about getting to know your body. The best way to get to know your body is to move naturally, explore as you move, and get comfortable in all kinds of exploration. When you get familiar with how your body feels, you can accomplish anything you can feel your way through with ease.

FACING CHALLENGES WITH NATURAL MOVEMENT

Okay. Now that you've gotten the idea of what natural movement is, let's see if we can use it to take on some seriously challenging poses: handstand rocks, flying crow, and flying twisted crow.

Exploring challenging movements often brings up tension right away. When we find something hard to do, we often hold everything tight and wait for the discomfort to pass. Or we throw everything we have at it and power right through. But that's not how it has to be. If you move naturally, focusing on each moment and flowing with ease, you can accomplish things like a handstand—even if you think there's no possible way. And this is true for the rest of your life too. Whenever we face a challenge, it's best to be alert, calm, and clear. Again, practicing this outlook on the mat will help you bring it into your everyday life. Plus you'll end up doing some really cool-looking moves!

I know you may not believe me, but this process of natural movement and paying attention to the moment can take us to and beyond any movement we can imagine doing. When we forget about the goal of the pose or the move-ment, we can concentrate fully on the process and achieve more with less effort. This is when we really get in the zone or in the flow—however you want to label it. You can do anything you dream possible by getting into the pro-cess. So even if you just *know* you won't be able to do these poses, give them a shot. Just remember to tune in to your body and move how it feels good to move. You may not get these right away—or even for quite a while—but if you keep trying, you'll get 'em.

HANDSTAND ROCKS

All right! Here comes a fun one. Handstand rocks! This movement is so much more than that scary handstand. Sure, we'll move through that one, but we're going through the process of getting there and beyond "there" in handstand rocks. Why waste all the fun on just a handstand? The exploration is the excitement and will lead beyond one picture of a pose.

Something fun happens when we go upside down, and that something is different for all of us. For some, handstands are exciting and give a sense of freedom and joy. For some, handstands are the scariest thing in the world, a cause of anxiety or even sickness. We will explore all of that inside an internal experience of the physical practice of rocking. With this movement, the handstand becomes a hip opener, which is designed to help you feel open, at ease, and calm. When we add calm to this emotional—exciting or fear-inducing—experience, we gain a nice sense of grounding and safety in the process.

Another cool thing about handstand rocks is that it is designed to take you as far as you'd like to go. This process doesn't just end in a handstand with your legs straight up like a diver's. You can make that one of your stops along the way, but there are also endless possibilities to shapes and movements you can explore in your body with ease while we practice. This is the handstand that keeps on giving. Let's rock it!

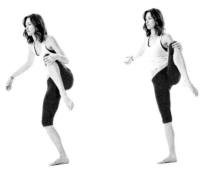

Start standing with one knee hugged gently toward your chest.
Soften your standing knee, and roll gently around in your hips.
Now you're movable—so let's move!

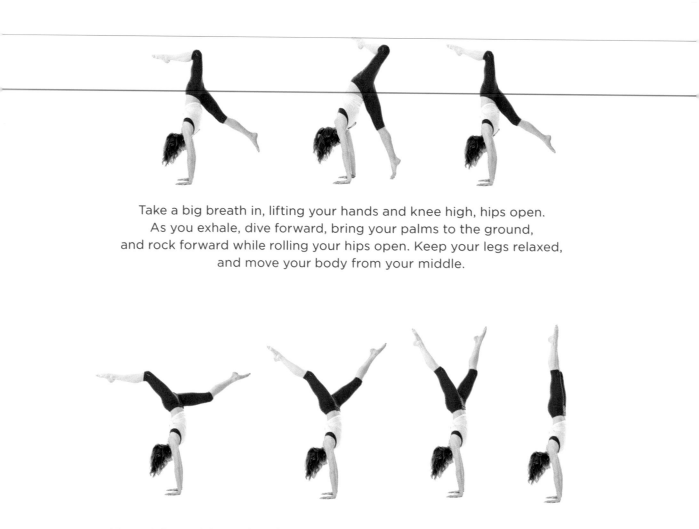

Take a big breath in, lifting your hands and knee high, hips open.
As you exhale, dive forward, bring your palms to the ground,
and rock forward while rolling your hips open. Keep your legs relaxed,
and move your body from your middle.

You might rock into a handstand, keeping one leg forward and one back,
both legs relaxed, knees bent, finding an easy balance. You might just rock
your hips forward while breathing in, putting weight into your arms as
you roll your hips open, and then rock gently back while breathing out,
relaxing your body so it's ready to rock again.

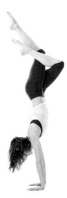

If you hold the balance, it's playtime!

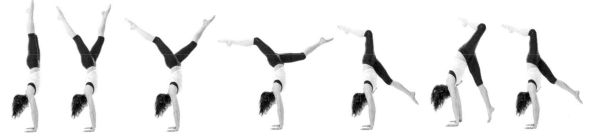

Stay relaxed enough in your body that it can find its own balance easily,
as you roll gently around in your hips. Maybe you stretch your legs
straight up, or split side to side, or wrap them around each other.

FLYING CROW

Don't be scared, but we're going to fly! This movement is simple when you approach the process with ease and have fun flowing through each moment. The great thing about flying crow is that it's a continuous movement, not a destination, so it's great for exploring your body and mind. The pictures are merely markers of possible places where you can take this. Your imagination is the only limitation to your actual destination. Stay easy and enjoy the ride here.

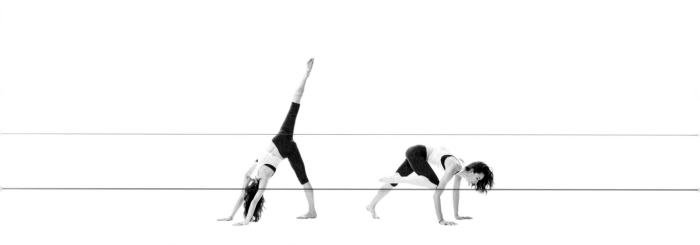

From down dog split, right leg high, take a big inhale to
open your hips, then easy exhale to bend and arc your knee high
around to your upper right arm.

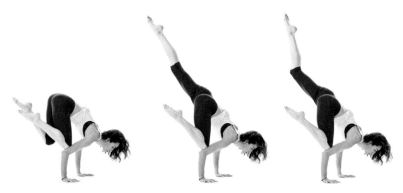

Gently bend your right arm to make a little shelf for your knee, then look forward
and lean forward into a balance. If it's easy for you to lean into this, you can
soften your back knee and pull it toward you, gently lifting your back foot off the
ground, no jumping required! You can lift that leg high if that feels good to you.
You're flying!

Ease out of it by rebending your left knee and lowering your foot softly back
to the ground; then take a big inhale to pull your right leg high to a down dog split.
If your back foot doesn't lift easily, no problem! Just soften your back knee and
roll gently around in your hips, getting to know your body all around the pose.
Try lifting your hips a little higher, by bringing your back foot in a bit closer. Keep
exploring gently in every direction you can move, and soon enough even the
hardest poses are no problem at all! Now try it on the other side.

FLYING TWISTED CROW

Now that you've played around a bit with flying crow, the twisted version will be like a nice breeze carrying you through. This movement is great to get your whole body moving in all directions. It's a nice twist that feels great, a feel-good hip opener, and a great moment of fun flying. When you move naturally with ease, it becomes simple and light. Try it out and enjoy!

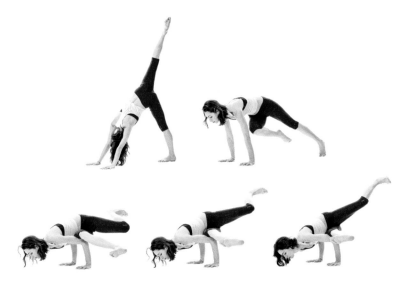

From down dog split, right leg high, take a big inhale to open your hips; then easy exhale to drop your knee down and across your body, letting the knee bend as it moves. Bend your elbows to make a little shelf for your upper right thigh on your upper left arm. You can rest your right toes on the ground as you move into this; then look forward and lean forward into the balance. If it's easy for you to lean into this, your back foot will lift gently off the ground. Now you can play around, maybe by extending both legs straight. To come out of this, soften both knees as you gently lower your right toes, then left toes to the ground. Keep both knees soft as you press into your palms, and inhale to lift your hips high and right leg back through and open to a down dog split. If it's not so easy to lift into the balance, there's plenty to do with your feet on the ground! Just keep your knees soft, and roll gently around in your hips with your right thigh resting on your left upper arm. Get to know your body this way, and hard things will become easy soon enough! Now give it all a try on the other side.

PRINCIPLES OF MOVEMENT

Now that you understand what natural movement is, we're ready to dive in to two movement principles that support you in getting directly into the flow. These are "the magic in three" and "go back to go forward." These principles are designed to inspire natural movement because they complement our nature and work with what we respond to as emotional beings. They are based in things that give us comfort and provide a foundation for us to feel great and achieve amazing things.

In Strala classes we aim to incorporate these ideas into our routines—and you can do the same if you get to the point where you are creating your own. Moving through a class is designed to feel like a day at the beach, like an afternoon observing the forest, or like living inside a lovely piece of poetry or music. So much of what we respond to and are inspired by comes directly from patterns in nature, which, of course, are the patterns of who we are.

THE MAGIC IN THREE

I think I first heard it on *Sesame Street* that three is the magic number. We find it everywhere. On your mark, get set, go before a race. One, two, three before a picture. There is something special and safe about the space that a count to three creates. It gets us ready. Really ready, and then we go! Of course, there is lots of symbolism in our world with threes. Body/mind/spirit, Father/Son/Holy Ghost, three counts in the waltz, third time's a charm—it's with us everywhere. Perhaps this is why it feels so comfortable to us.

When it comes to the Strala routines, we often start movements in sets of three. One cycle gets things moving. A second is nice for opening even more. And a third feels familiar and safe and gives a sense of completion and closure. We take three breaths in the beginning of class—three long inhales and exhales all together. On the first breath, it's like jumping in the pool. An instant sense of refreshment floods the body and mind. By the second breath, we're feeling more open and calm. During the third, a sense of connectedness takes over, and we're in the flow. The repetition and familiarity all add to our ability to move naturally.

Progression and repetition happen often in sets of three, as well. Say we go for a high lunge and back to down dog. The next round we revisit the high lunge and go for a twist, come right back to high lunge, repeat that twice more, and continue on with a warrior 2 and then something else that feels great. We have a more expansive and complex movement phrase now, but the repetition in threes brings familiarity and comfort, which helps us achieve the movement with ease. Adding on to a movement that we've tried out on a previous round gives more familiarity and ease to something that could be more challenging and uneasy with only one try and then forgotten about. Letting it all soak in, enjoying a day at the park, feeling the cool breeze across our faces, it's all a familiar dance of repetition and familiarity.

Once a set of three is established, we often move to a familiar moment breathed through once. If everything were organized in sets of threes, the threes wouldn't feel as special or as useful as they are when they're sprinkled in a natural setting with sets of one. Theme and variation carry us through music, poetry, art, and nature. Having a phrase with a set of three, followed by a phrase gone through once, and followed up with a three-set phrase provides an enjoyable rhythmic drive to the practitioner. Almost as you would rise with joy for your favorite part of a piece of music you know is coming up while you're thoroughly enjoying the present melody, the pattern and rhythm of the piece uplifts you, setting you in a time-stand-still zone of total flow. Designing movement phrases is like designing poetry. We learn a language, and then organize the structure to ignite emotion. I'll guide you through a simple movement phrase that happens first in threes and then ones so you can try it on for size.

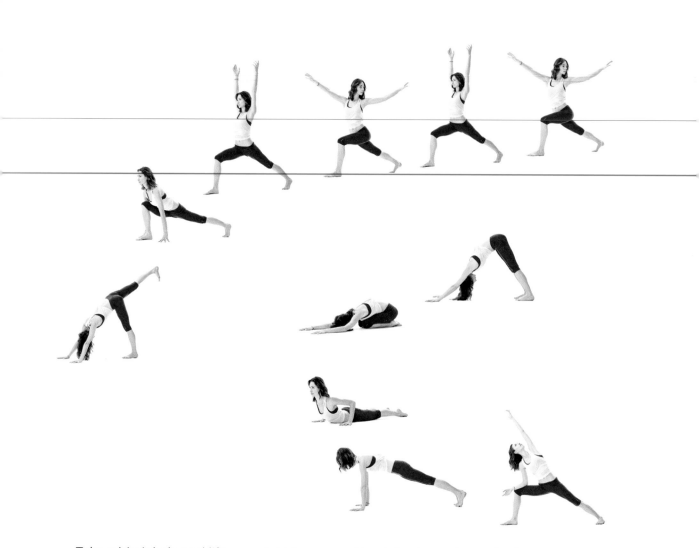

Take a big inhale and lift your right leg up and back to down dog split. Open up your hips and shoulders if that feels nice. Step your foot on through to a low lunge. Press down through your legs, take a big inhale, and lift up to high lunge. Exhale and twist to your front leg; let your arms open wide out to your sides. Take a big inhale and lift back to high lunge. Twice more just like that. Big exhale, easy twist to your front leg. Big inhale back to your high lunge. Big exhale, easy twist. Big inhale up and back and open into warrior 2. Spin your back heel down, open your arms out to your sides, and sink your hips. Soften in here for a moment. Take a big inhale and lift your hips and arms up. Exhale and soften back to warrior 2. Repeat twice more.

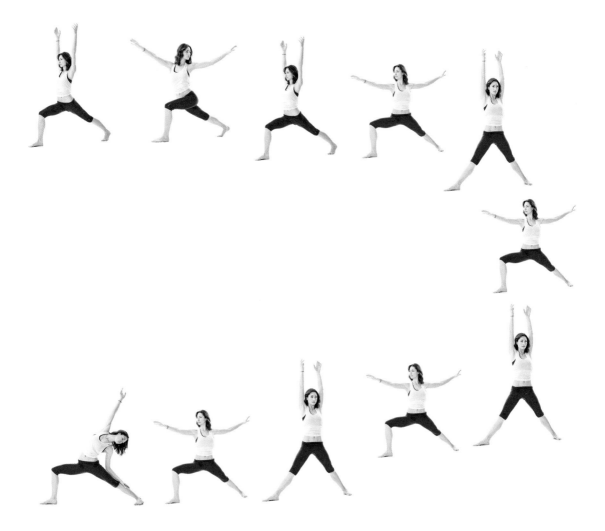

From warrior 2 take a big inhale and tip your torso back to reverse warrior. Take an easy exhale and tip forward to extended side angle. Roll your torso open and move how it feels good to you here. Plant your palms on the ground and step back to a plank position. Soften your knees to the ground and sink your hips toward the ground, swaying your torso gently side to side. If this doesn't feel nice on your lower back, soften your elbows a bit more and lower your torso toward the ground, opening up your upper and middle back a bit. Keep your knees on the ground and shift your hips back to sit on your heels for child's pose. Rest your torso on the ground and hang here for a couple breaths. When you are ready, come onto all fours. Spread your fingers wide like you are digging into wet sand, tuck your toes, take a big inhale, and lift your hips up and back to down dog.

Try the movements on your other side.

How did that feel? Did you feel the opening and settling into the moves because of the use of threes? Did you feel how the twisting three times to the right was essentially preparation for opening to warrior 2? This set of three was designed to allow you to settle into warrior 2 for a few breaths and feel really nice and spacious. The repetitive twisting and opening movement winds you up in a way to fully enjoy opening up even more into warrior 2.

So as you can see, the theory of threes plays a role in inspiring natural movement. When you're working through the routines in this book, you may notice some of this happening, but more important, if you start creating your own routines based on what feels good to you, you can incorporate this idea.

GO BACK TO GO FORWARD

Another fun principle of movement is go back to go forward. This idea, which calls for you to move in one direction in order to head in another, creates physical and emotional space and feels expansive. Go back to go forward, go down to go up, go left to go right—all of these are ideas where opposites initiate direction.

From a practical standpoint, moving gently in one direction before heading in another creates ease of balance in movement. A wave curls back and up before rushing into shore and curls back and up again to repeat another rush. No two waves are alike. When we apply this principle of movement to our own bodies and lives, we stay in balance by moving easily in all directions. If we were to move only in the direction we wanted to go without gently dipping into the opposite, we'd end up with something forced and jammed up. The breath and space go missing.

This concept may sound a bit familiar because it has already been incorporated into the work we've been doing. Lifting up to create space helps you settle more deeply into warrior 2. Just as twisting in one direction helps loosen moves in the other direction. Moving in the opposite direction often helps you move more fully in the direction you'd like. It creates ease by creating balance.

JUST GOING FORWARD

Moving through reverse warrior to get to extended side angle is an example of going back to go forward. You created space in your body for the forward movement to happen by first tipping back. If you'd like to see what it's like when you don't do this, come into warrior 2, stay for a few deep breaths, and then tip forward into extended side angle and stay for a few deep breaths. Come back to warrior 2. Repeat this a few times to get the full experience. It won't feel like the worst movement in the world, but it won't feel as free and open as it does when you do the movement with the spaciou s tip back before tipping forward.

❈

Let's give it a try. In the routine you're about to do, you go down to go up, back to go forward, and left to go right. Once you allow yourself to soften, move easily, and get in the flow, you'll start to see there isn't much difference between the simple and the challenging. This is the place where things get really exciting. Enjoy!

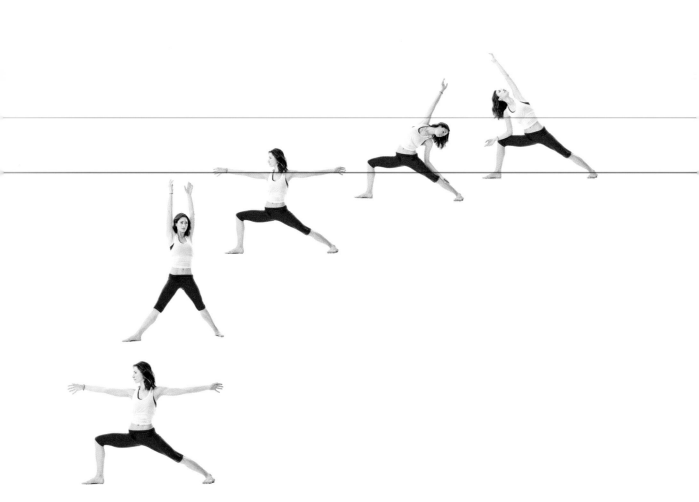

Take a nice, wide stance, a few feet apart. Turn your right toes toward your right, left toes slightly in. Take a big inhale and open your arms out to your sides. Exhale and soften into warrior 2. Sink your hips low, bending your front knee over your front foot. Take a few breaths here, letting the inhale lift you up softly, and the exhale settle you back in.

Take a big inhale and lift your hips and arms up. Exhale and soften back to warrior 2.

From warrior 2 take a big inhale and tip your torso back to reverse warrior. Let your hips lift naturally as you tip back. As you exhale bring your torso forward to extended side angle. Rest your right forearm on your right thigh and open your left arm up overhead. Roll your torso open a bit if that feels nice for you.

In extended side angle you are free to move a bit easily, according to how it feels best for you. Try pressing down gently through your feet and down from your forearm on your thigh to open up space to roll your torso open.

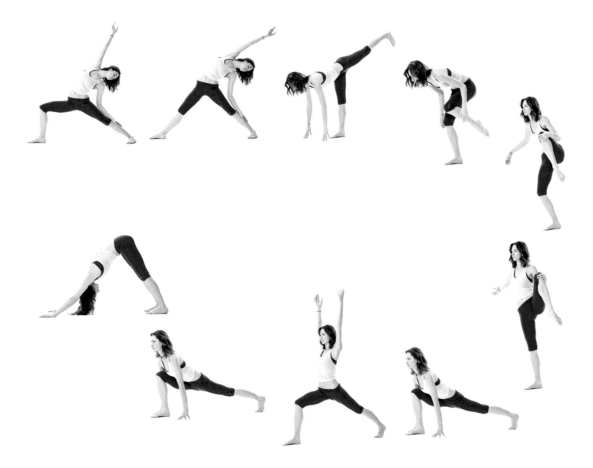

From extended side angle take a big inhale, lifting up through warrior 2 and tipping back to reverse warrior. Sweep through from here. Soften your knees as you crawl your torso forward toward your front foot. Crawl your fingertips on the ground out in front of you. As your weight comes onto your front leg, curl your back leg in, rounding your back naturally, curling into a soft ball. Take a big inhale, extend your back leg behind you, and open your torso forward into warrior 3.

From warrior 3, soften your knees, round your back, and roll up to hug your left shin into your chest. Roll your shin around a bit to open the hips while keeping your standing leg soft for balance.

Soften your knees and step your left leg long behind you to low lunge. Press down through your legs and take a big inhale to lift up to high lunge, lifting your hips and arms up. Exhale and soften back to low lunge, pressing your hands on the ground on either side of your front foot. Press down through your hands and find your way back to down dog, either stepping right to it or moving through a flow that feels great for you.

This routine included a lot of going back to go forward and up to go down. You likely experienced the difference between incorporating the opposite movement if you tried my suggestion in the "Just Going Forward" box. But that wasn't the only time we used this idea.

Moving between warrior 2 and warrior 2 lift is an expression of up to go down. We lift and create space by breathing in and letting the body go along for the ride. We can use the power of the breath to simply breathe in, or to fuel the body to lift up. With warrior 2 lift, the breath fuels the body, and the whole body lifts. The movement is continuous just like a wave that curls up and rolls in. There is never a moment of stop and decide. There is only flow.

In extended side angle, pressing down on your feet and forearm is another way you go down to go up. It's less visible in a big movement, but you should be able to feel it while moving through. It's incredibly useful for creating room in the body, igniting the relaxation response, and stabilizing balance through easy movement.

We went back to go forward in the reverse warrior to sweep through to warrior 3. This created space and ease of balance for the one-legged warrior 3. By going up and in to go out and down, we realize that movement is circular instead of linear.

Finally, we practiced down to go up with low lunge to high lunge, which gave fresh life to the movement.

The design of moving circularly is for you to feel capable, light, and easy as you cultivate strength, balance, and awareness in your body, mind, and life. When we move in opposites, we are able to approach challenges with ease, and we realize the expansion is limitless.

A LITTLE MORE OF A CHALLENGE

If you're up for a challenge, let's play around with balance on one leg, balance upside down, and putting it all together. We prepared for the handstand by rolling around in the hips and belly while balancing on one leg. Handstand is simply the reverse of this movement while rolling down and shifting the weight on the hands. This movement is another example of going down to go up and in to go out. Everything is happening all together all at the same time.

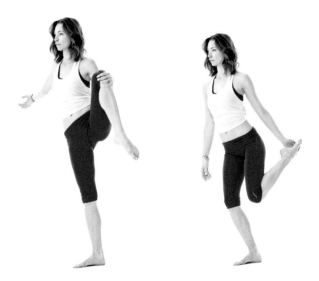

Let's take the one-legged balances another step. From shin hug, relax your knee so it points toward the ground. Grab ahold of the inside of your left foot with your left hand. Soften your standing knee. Let your whole body relax. Just as it's important to go down to go up, back to go forward, it is also important to soften before you move. If you move from a place of tension, you're very likely to stay tense and you'll probably tip over in a frustrated heap, raising your stress levels. When you move from a place of ease, you stay easy and are able to explore new possibilities, and if you tip, you tip with ease, continue to ignite the relaxation response, expand your comfort zone safely, and enjoy the ride.

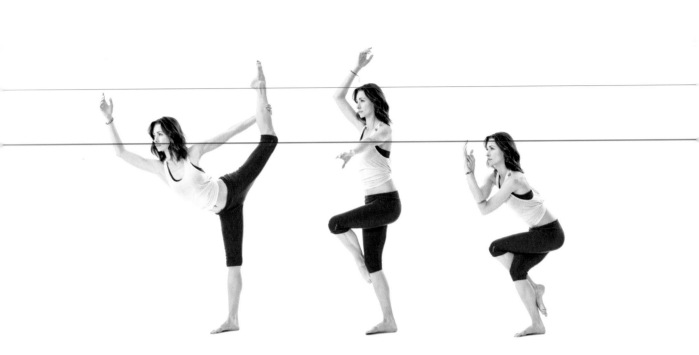

Take a big inhale and press your left shin into your hand behind you. Lift your right arm up for balance. As you exhale soften everything, release your shin, bringing your legs in toward each other. Take a big inhale and lift up, opening your left leg out to your side and your arms out, as well. Exhale and wrap your left leg over your right into eagle and your left arm under your right in front of you. Sink through your hips and gently lift up through your fingertips. Here is your easy eagle movement! The secret of embodying our eagle friends is, of course, in staying easy and soft as you move and sinking as you lift. There is the down to go up. The wrapping motion is big, expansive, and circular, sweeping into balance. If the wrap with one leg off the ground feels unstable, you can always press the toes of your wrapped leg on the ground for more support. There is always a way to back off and feel more stable. Stability and ease are always the priority to the movement. They are the qualities that direct the relaxation response to turn on, the body to strengthen and gain a healthy range of motion, the intuition to strengthen, and the emotional feeling of limitless expansion to crack wide-open.

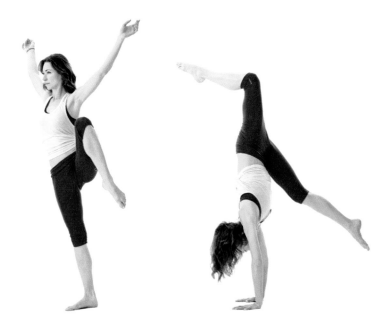

Ready for more? Let's go upside down. From eagle, take a big inhale and unravel your arms and legs, lifting your arms up overhead. Take a gentle dive up and over your standing leg and plant your hands on the ground with some strength in your arms. Rock gently forward onto your arms, getting your hips over your shoulders. Roll around in your hips and belly as you rock. As you rock back, exhale and relax. Roll through this a few times with your breath and enjoy. Avoid jumping, abandoning your breath-body connection, and stiffening up as you move. These are typical pitfalls of handstand exploration that usually lead to crashing, and even when they lead to sticking your handstand, they come along with a big dose of stress for your system. Enjoy rocking forward and back, transferring your weight onto your arms. A little hop is okay, and easy on your body, but feel your way around; explore here. Enjoy the process, and you will reach your destination with ease.

Right there we explored down to go up with pressing into the arms and rocking forward and back. Every soften back is the down, and every breath in to rock is the up. Keep exploring with the down to go up wave ideas in mind, and enjoy the ride.

When you've had enough handstand exploration on that side, let's even out this movement phrase. Soften your knees and find your way back to down dog. Gently walk your feet up to your hands, roll up, hugging your right shin, and go for the other side. Stay easy in your body and mind as you move through the challenges. There is no need to achieve the positions. The movements will get easier with practice.

REFLECTION MOMENT

Now that we're in the luxurious, natural, continuous movement, it's a good opportunity to take this a step further and consider how this practice applies to life. We all have moments and phases where we feel stuck, and moments where we feel the joy of being in our natural flow. I encourage you to take a moment to reflect and take in the concepts and how they apply to life.

Explore however it works best for you to internalize and reflect on your experience. Here are a few questions to get you going:

☆　Are there moments in my life where I feel disconnected from my natural self?

☆　Do I feel mostly out of the flow or in the flow of my life?

☆　When I'm doing _____ things come easily for me.

☆　How do I feel when I'm in my natural flow?

☆　When I'm thinking about _____ I feel stuck and tense.

☆　Do I feel more connected to my internal or external experience of life?

☆　Do I worry about proving my value to people and end up performing life instead of acting how I really feel?

☆　Do I move easily in my life with a sense of comfort and joy, or is getting around rushed and clunky feeling?

☆　Would I like to be more connected to my natural way of being in the world?

☆　Do I think a physical practice of natural movement can shift how I deal with living a life aligned with my natural self?

Living from our natural sense of self puts us right in the center of our ability to be effective and enjoy what we put our efforts into. When we feel out of the flow, we are moving from a place of fear and insecurity. Our movements and actions are clunky, out of sorts, and frazzled. When we are in the flow, we are moving from a place of joy and purpose. Our movements and actions are soft, gracious, and peaceful. We accomplish challenges with ease, and we enjoy the balance and natural rhythm of life. We all experience moments of flow and moments of clunk. The secret is in realizing when the clunky is happening and deciding to take action to bring ourselves back to the flow, where our natural, amazing self is waiting to come out and play.

CONTINUOUS MOVEMENT

The nature of movement is circular and continuous. Nature never stops breathing or moving. It simply slows and quickens, changing quality and mood seamlessly. We are the same when we remember to move naturally. When we forget, we hold our breath, wait for the challenge to be over, or tough it out, powering through in a way that doesn't work well, stressing ourselves out in the process. Having the awareness of being human comes along with the joy and burden of the possibilities of making choices. When we choose well, we flourish, grow, and expand. When we choose poorly, we get in our own way with our thoughts and stress. We move in a way that is stiff and tense, collecting blocks in our bodies, minds, and lives. How we move is a reflection of how we feel about ourselves. We have a big opportunity available every day to practice how we would like to be by practicing how we move.

Natural movement is luxurious, effective, continuous, and poetic. We can contemplate, reflect, express, and practice this concept. We can observe it in nature by watching a tree sway in the breeze. We can practice simply by drawing our attention to our breath, watching it come and go as we inhale and exhale. We can move this practice into our physical world by letting our breath fuel our movement, continuously lifting and softening our bodies as we breathe. We can move essentially in any direction we can imagine if we let the breath do all the lifting for us; we are simply along for the ride.

Now that we are revved up, let's take a big, deep inhale and a long, easy, expansive exhale, and begin. Start where you are with each moment and you'll always end up somewhere surprising and amazing. Remember—if you can breathe, you can do yoga, so you've got this.

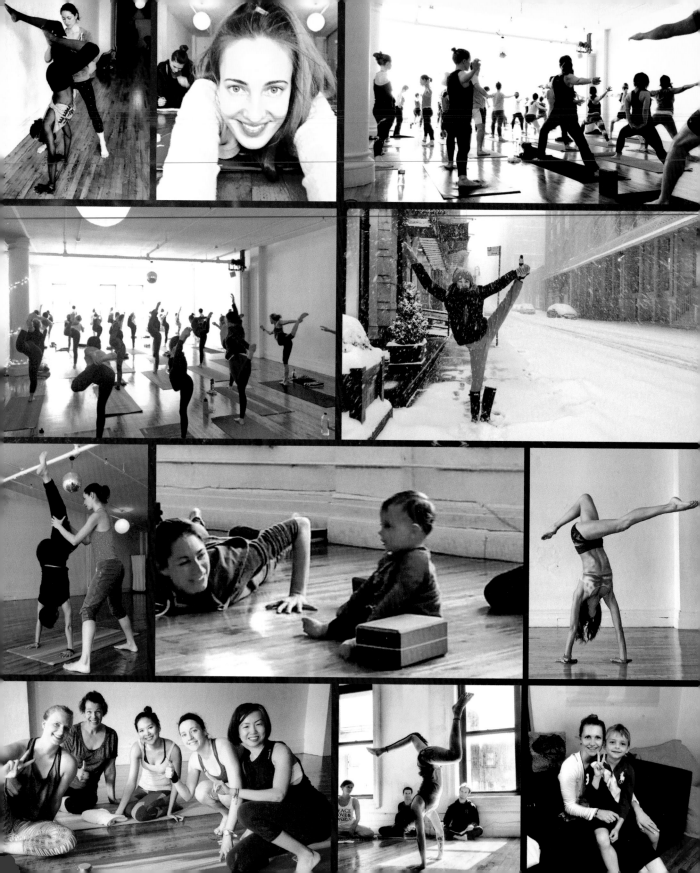

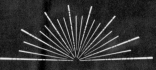

CHAPTER 5

SET UP

cultivating
a regular practice

NOW that we've explored the concepts of moving with ease physically and emotionally and tried them out in a few short practices and ideas, we're ready to infuse this practice into life. Yoga and meditation—your regular practice of paying attention to your breath—will make you feel fantastic from the inside out!

CREATE YOUR SPACE

The first thing we can do to get this sorted is create some physical space in your life to instill this positive change. The great news is you don't need much space to practice or much equipment for that matter, either. The only room you need is enough to lie down flat, sit upright, and stand up tall. You can literally use the space next to your bed if that's all you have. If you have a more spacious living room—or some other room—that's great too. Take a moment to identify which space in your home would work best for you to practice regularly. If you have the choice, find a space that is simple and clear, has some natural light, and feels great to you. Warning: this experiment might start a larger project of clearing your living space to create room for you to feel great. I do this all the time, organizing and updating my surroundings to best suit my goal of feeling good.

Personally I thrive in simplicity and a minimal approach. The fewer things around me, the better I feel. I've had some of my favorite meditation and yoga practices in minimal spaces or, even better, out in nature—just me and the beauty of the earth around me. At home I have a cozy space for meditation in a corner snuggled between a couple of bookshelves and my big bag of yarn for knitting. There's also a rocking chair nearby with a few memorable and colorful gifts from people I have met on my travels. A nice spherical glow lamp lights up this corner, and I have a contemplative piece of art hanging on the wall above. I love this corner because it has a strong sense of learning and reflection for me, and it just feels really good. The bright colors from the yarn make it easy to be inspired, and the books that live on my shelves call out to be read when I locate myself near them daily. It's an area of beauty, growth, and enrichment, and that's why I chose this place for meditation. When I'm traveling I choose a place in my hotel room or guest room that is simple and feels good. The place doesn't have to be much, and the things in it and nearby aren't that important, but the more attention you start to pay to how you feel, the more your exterior will start to reflect how you want to feel and be a positive and clear environment for you to cultivate a great life.

One suggestion I give to everyone who is trying to create a home practice is to avoid clutter because it can be a distraction, and it surrounds you with a feeling of chaos. If you have a few meaningful things in your space, that's great, but keep it minimal.

Also, there is no need to search for or purchase stuff to add value to your space. A home that comes together naturally over time is a nice reflection of your life, and this will help put you at ease. Creating a peaceful home helps you maintain an inspired internal world. Your practice is internal and personal, and most of it can happen with your eyes closed. The more you fill your space, the less space you have around you. It's a nice concept to keep space open, even when you accumulate things for your space naturally.

YOUR GEAR

Something I've always loved about the practice of yoga and meditation is how little you need to practice anywhere. Literally you simply need yourself and the ability to breathe. This is a fantastic start. It's possible to practice without a mat, blanket, props, or even specific yoga clothes. As long as you're comfortable and able to move your body a bit, you're in great shape. When I travel I rarely pack a yoga mat. I simply use the floor in my hotel room—or even the bed for simple practices. Even in the tiniest of rooms, there's enough space. It's a very nice reminder that everything we need rests inside.

With all that simplicity in mind, you may still want to gift yourself a yoga mat for support in your practice. There is a wide range of yoga mats geared toward all kinds of practices. If you sweat a lot, there are thicker mats made of rubber that are wonderful to keep your hands and feet where you want them. There are towels with little sticky bottoms to also put over your mat if you tend to slide. This will help keep you steady. If you prefer more padding for your knees, hips, and back, there are mats that are a little thicker and squishier, and these are fantastic for comfort.

I sweat a lot, but not so much from my hands and feet that I need a sweat-resistant mat or towel. I like a little cushion, so I go for a mat that has a little squish, but not so much that it's a mattress. In all honesty I'm not that picky; I'll use whatever is around. And if there's nothing around, I'm fine with the floor. There are so many fun mats out there to pick from. Many now come with inspirational messages, exciting patterns, and colors of all sorts. Most sporting goods, athletic-focused, and yoga stores carry a few different varieties of mats. You can usually ask to "try out" a mat at a store and feel it for your preferred amount of softness and traction. If you're traveling to and from a yoga studio or gym to practice, you might want to bring your own mat with you, but most studios have them available to either borrow or rent. My biggest piece of advice is don't stress about it. You aren't going to pick a mat that hurts you. And if you aren't in love with your mat, you can always get a new one. They aren't crazy expensive.

CREATING A REGULAR PRACTICE

Okay! You've got your space set up, and you're ready to go. Now what? Ha! Believe me, I know it can feel overwhelming when you're trying to change your life. But the good news is that you're already on the path. So my suggestion is to start slowly. Creating a permanent healthy change in life doesn't generally start with a sudden jolt. It starts with baby steps. Yes, an initial push can get you going, but most people burn out if they don't ease into things. So before you start with a plan to do 30 minutes of meditation followed by an hour of yoga every day, really think about what you will be able to maintain. Maybe you'll simply want to do 10 minutes of meditation today. Then tomorrow 10 minutes of meditation and 10 minutes of yoga. You honestly have to figure out what's right for you.

In Part Two of the book, I've broken down several practices for you. These routines are based on classes we teach at Strala. They are open to anyone, any age, any body type, any background or level of experience. The routines are designed to deliver a clear process of moving with ease and connecting to yourself. Let yourself feel good in the movements as you explore. Each inhale lifts and expands you. Every exhale softens and moves you a bit farther. One always comes after another, so you're always right where you need to be, connected with your breath. The Strala concept is designed to make you feel great the entire time. I hope you enjoy an oceanic wavelike ride that connects you to your intuition and creativity, and energizes every cell of your body, creating space for your awesomeness to radiate everywhere you go.

If you want more of a challenge, or more of a relaxing moment, always feel free to add more or back off, following how you feel. Feeling great the entire time is the priority. Stay easy and enjoy!

Pick your practice based on how you want to feel. When you want a boost of steam to get things going in your body and mind, go for ENERGIZE. When you feel frazzled and stressed and want to calm and focus things, move through RELAX. When you want something ultrasoft to hit the reset button, enjoy GENTLE. When you want a little extra strength and fire in your middle, move through CORE. When you want a nice reset, I've got BASICS ready for you. Keep the focus on feeling and moving along easy with your breath to fully enjoy the practice and soak up all the benefits.

In addition to these Strala class routines, which are based on desired feeling, I've included one chapter of what I call "Target Practices." These are aimed at giving you some desired effect: To wake you up when you didn't get enough sleep. To detox you when you had a bit too much fun the previous night—or month. To help you wind down when you need to rest but feel too chaotic. To dissolve stress when the tension is holding its grasp on you. To sleep better so you can have a restful and productive day.

If you want even more instruction to help make yoga and meditation part of your life, I have laid out a 7-day jump start and a 30-day guide in Part Three of the book. Both of these will take some of the work of deciding what to do out of your hands. But they're not the only way to do this. You have to feel into yourself. Tap into your intuition. You'll be able to figure out what you want. Just make sure to do something.

IT'S NOT EASY, BUT IT'S EASYGOING

The fun and effectiveness of Strala rests in the "how" of the practice. The movements are soft and continuous. You'll accomplish more than you might think you can—and with less effort. It's joyful and fun because of the ingredients that you apply, like the breath-body connection, the reminder to feel, and natural movement. It's not important what movements you can or cannot do. What matters is how you do everything you do. It's not always easy, but it's easygoing. When you direct yourself to move in the flow of "easygoing," your experience spontaneously shifts to joyful, relaxed, focused, and calm. Stay easy and enjoy!

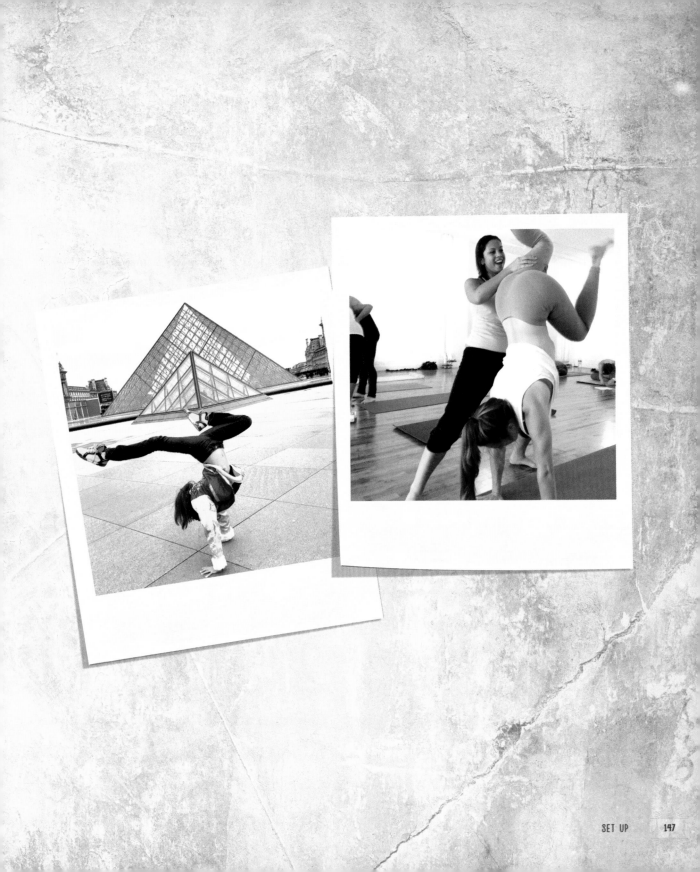

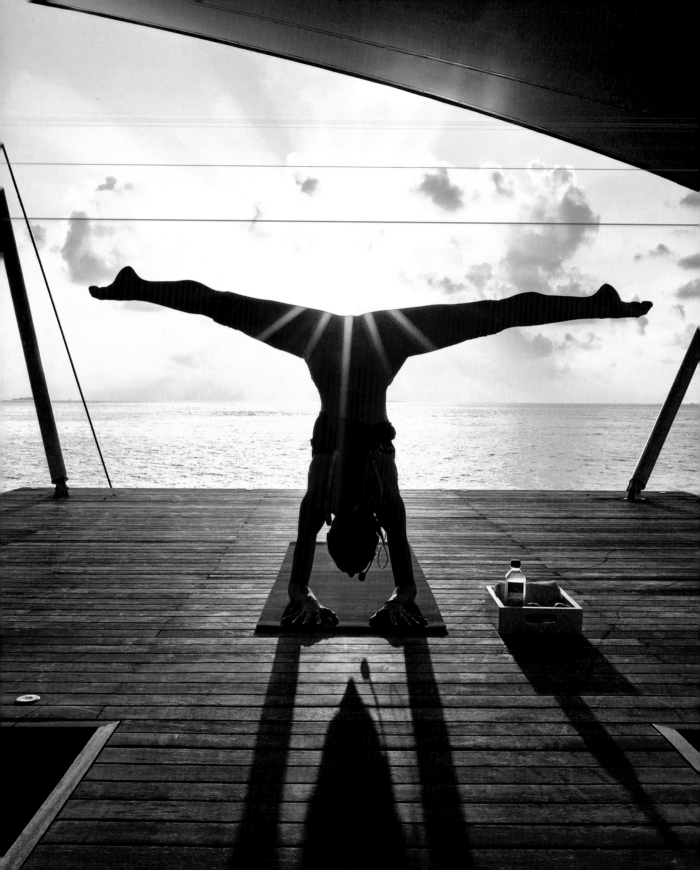

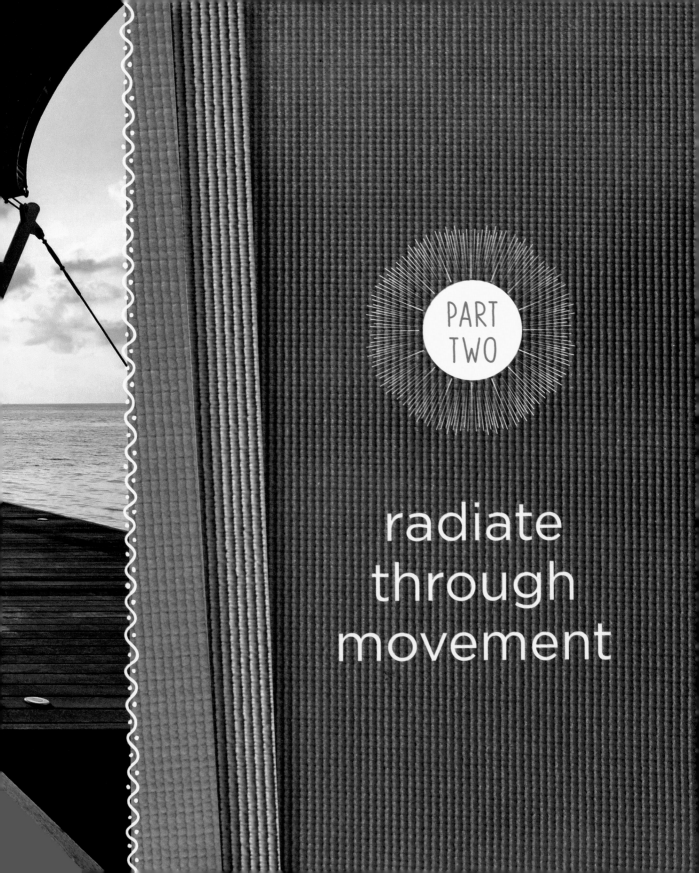

PART
TWO

radiate
through
movement

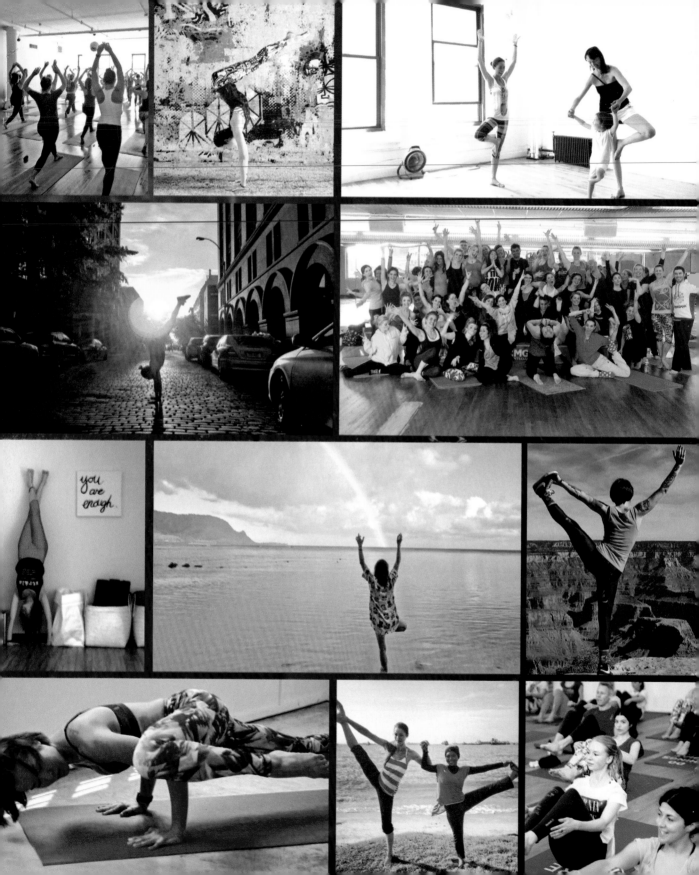

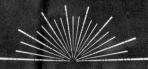

CHAPTER 6

ENERGIZE

This practice is designed to invigorate your body and mind while resting your attention calmly on your breath. When you're done, you'll feel awake, revitalized, and supercreative! There are a few challenging movements in the routine, so remember to keep things easy in your body and back off if something doesn't feel great for you today. Breathe deeply and enjoy!

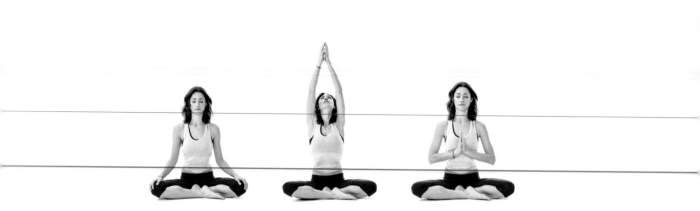

Start sitting, however you are comfortable. Close your eyes and rest your attention on your breath. If you notice your attention shifting, see if you can guide it right back to your breath.

Take a big inhale and lift your arms up overhead. Close your eyes, bring your palms together, and bring your thumbs to your heartbeat. Soften here for a moment. Take a big inhale through your nose. Long exhale out through your mouth. Twice more like that. Big inhale, long exhale. One more time. Big inhale, long exhale. When you are ready, gently relax your hands back on your thighs.

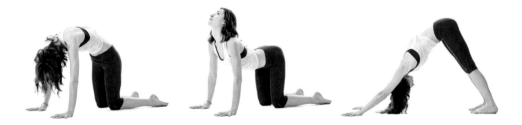

Staying soft and easy in your body, come onto all fours. Start to move a bit with your breath, moving your torso side to side, round and round, and forward and back, however feels good for you. When you're ready, tuck your toes, take a big inhale, and lift your hips up and back to down dog. Move around a bit here how it feels good for you to get comfortable and open up a bit.

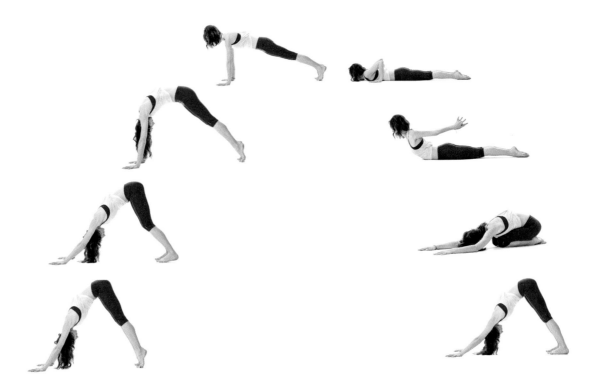

Take a big inhale and lift up on your tippy toes. Exhale and relax back. Twice more just like that, big inhale and lift, easy exhale and soften. One more time, big inhale and lift, easy exhale and soften. Tuck your chin and roll out into plank pose. Sway around here a bit if that feels nice. When you're ready, take a big inhale and lift your hips up and back to down dog. Once more just like that, tuck your chin and round out into plank. This time, soften your elbows and lower down to your belly. Interlace your hands behind you and lift up a bit, swaying side to side, however feels good for you. When you're ready, soften back to your belly. Press your palms on the ground under your shoulders. Keep your knees on the ground, shift your hips back to child's pose. Rest here for a moment. When you're ready, lift your hips, tuck your toes, and lift back into down dog.

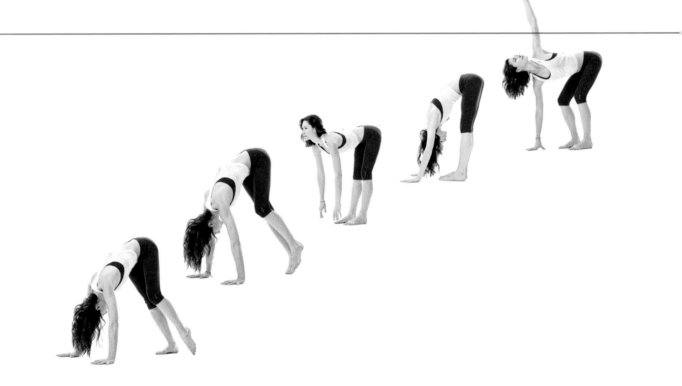

Take an easy walk up to your hands. Let your hands move if that feels
good, freeing up some space. Come into easy standing forward bend. If
you'd like, soften your knees to make some space for your hamstrings.
Relax your head and neck and breathe here for a bit. Soften your knees,
press your right fingertips on the ground, take a big inhale, and open your
body to your left, extending your left arm up. Gaze up if that feels nice.
Exhale and come through the middle and go for the other side, pressing
your left fingertips on the ground and opening your body to your right,

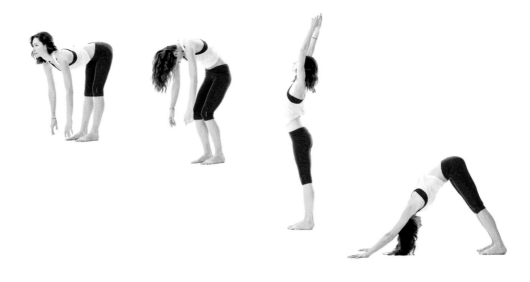

extending your right arm up. Gaze up if that feels nice. When you're ready, exhale and come to center. Keeping your head and neck soft, roll up to stand one notch at a time. When you make it up, take a big inhale and float your arms out and up. Easy exhale and round back into standing forward bend. Go for that twice more with your breath rounding up and down softly. When you're ready, plant your palms and find your way back to down dog, stepping or moving how it feels great to you.

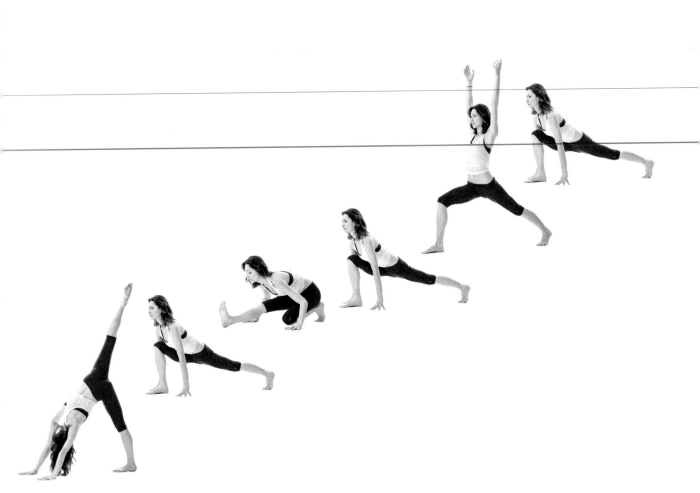

Take a big inhale and lift your right leg up and back to down dog split. Open your hips if that feels nice. Exhale and step your foot through to low lunge. Ease your back knee to the ground. Keeping your fingertips on the ground for support, shift your hips back toward your back heel, relaxing your torso over your front leg. Let your torso shift and drift side to side, however it feels good for you. When you're ready, crawl yourself back to low lunge. Keeping your fingertips on the ground for support, tuck your back toes and lift your hips up while relaxing your torso over your front leg. Keep your knees soft to take any tension out of the hamstrings and let your torso sway a bit to open up. When you're ready, sink your hips back to your low lunge, take a big inhale, and lift up to high lunge, lifting your hips and arms, and then

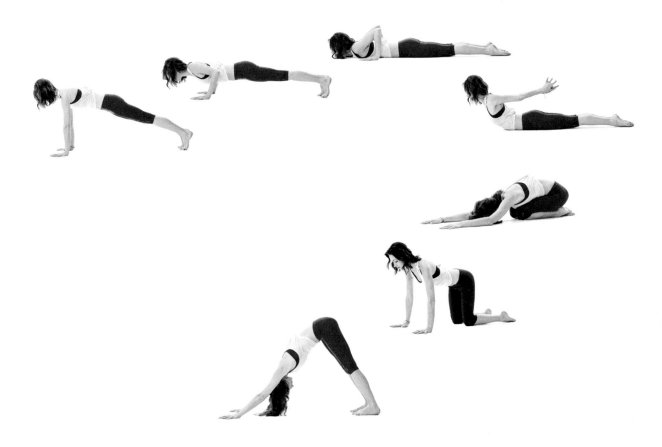

exhale back to low lunge and plant your palms on the ground on either side of your front foot. Step back to plank, soften your elbows, and lower down to your belly. Interlace your hands behind you and lift up a bit. Sway a little side to side, however it feels good for you. When you're ready, soften back to your belly. Press your palms on the ground next to your chest, and, keeping your knees on the ground, shift your hips to your heels to relax in child's pose. Hang here for a few breaths and when you're ready, come back onto all fours, spread your fingers wide, tuck your toes, take a big inhale, and lift your hips up and back to down dog. Soften here.

Repeat the movement phrase on the left side. Stay easy with your breath.

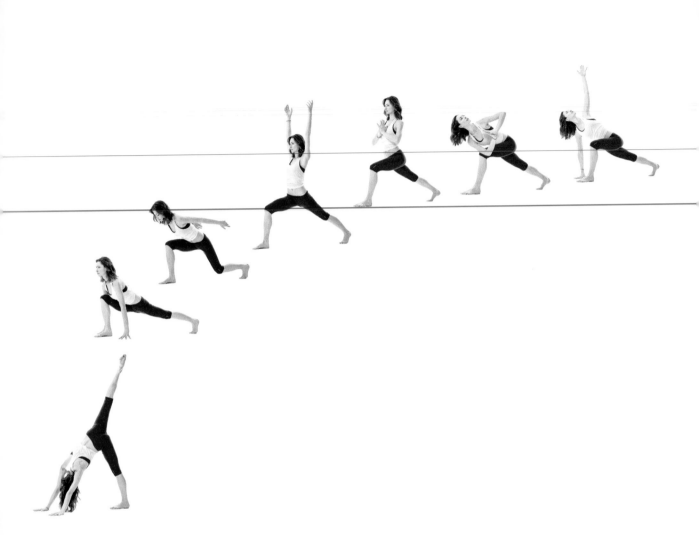

Take a big inhale and lift your right leg up to down dog split. Open your hips if that feels nice. Exhale and step your foot through to low lunge. Press down through your legs and inhale up into high lunge, lifting your hips and arms. Bring your palms together, exhale, and soften, bringing your thumbs to your heartbeat. Take a big inhale to lift up a bit. Exhale and twist toward your left side, bringing your right elbow outside your left thigh. Hang here for a few moments.

When you're ready, open your arms, bringing your right fingertips to the ground and your left arm up. Gaze upward if you'd like. When you're ready, bring the fingertips of both hands to the ground on either side of your front foot. Lift your hips up and soften your torso over your front leg. Sway here to open up for a bit. Spin your back heel down and open your torso toward your left side into a triangle. Open your left arm up and gaze

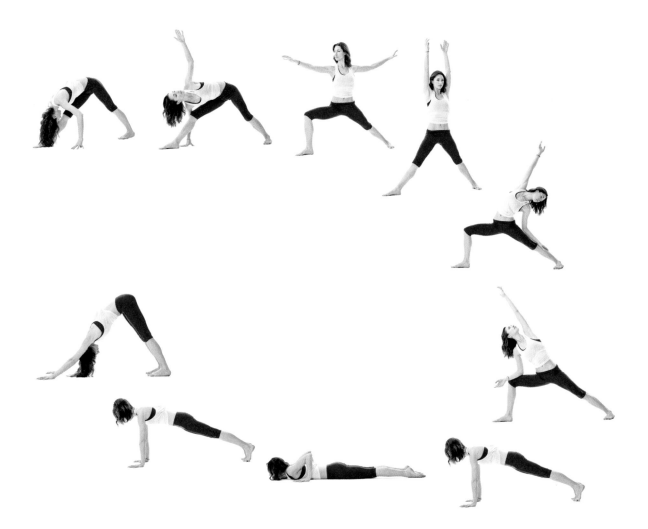

upward if that feels nice. Soften your knees, reach your top arm back, press down through your legs, and lift your hips up and your arms overhead.

Soften into warrior 2, bending your front knee over your front foot and relaxing your arms out to your sides. Take a big inhale and lift your hips and arms overhead. Soften back to warrior 2. Take a big inhale and tip back to reverse warrior, sliding your back hand gently down your back leg and your front arm overhead. Tip forward into extended side angle, pressing your top forearm on your thigh and your opposite arm overhead. Roll your belly open if that feels good. Press your palms on the ground on either side of your front foot and step back to plank. Soften your elbows and lower down to your belly. Take a big inhale and press right up through plank and up and back to down dog. Soften here.

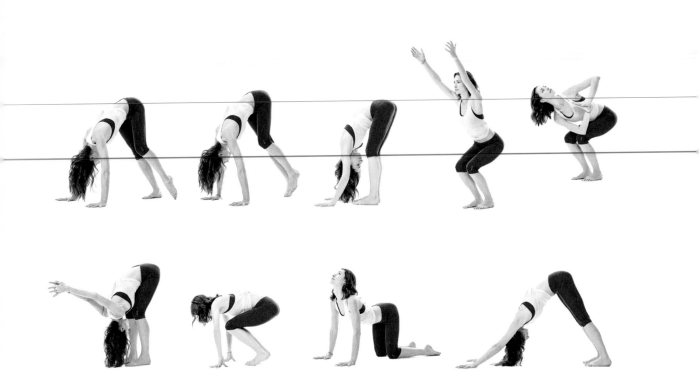

Walk your feet up to your hands one step at a time. Your hands can move also, to give yourself some room. Once you're up, relax your torso over your legs and hang here for a moment. Sway your torso a bit to open up. Bend your knees, sink your hips, take a big inhale, and lift your torso up into chair, lifting your arms overhead. Press your palms together in front of you, take an easy exhale, and twist toward your left, pressing your right elbow outside your knee and opening up to your left. Take a big inhale and come back to chair, lifting up in your hips a bit. Exhale and twist to your other side. Take a big inhale and come back to chair. Exhale and relax your torso over your legs, interlacing your hands behind you for a nice shoulder release. Sway a bit here if that feels nice. Plant your palms on the ground, shift your weight into your arms, and sink your hips to an easy squat. Bring your hands inside your legs and roll around here a bit to open your hips. If you'd like to play around with crow, plant your palms on the ground a bit in front of you, rock forward, bringing your knees onto the backs of your upper arms, and look forward. Exhale, rock back, and relax. Roll through this a few times with your breath rocking forward and back. Maybe one or both feet lift off the ground. Keep it easy. Don't jump or force your way into the movement. When you're ready, find your way back to down dog.

CROW
CRASH COURSE

There is a secret to having an effortless crow that involves looking into the future. Like any bird in flight, it's important to look where you'd like to go. Try gazing forward (not at the ground) a couple feet in front of you, or, as I like to lovingly guide, "into the future," because that's where you are headed for greatness!

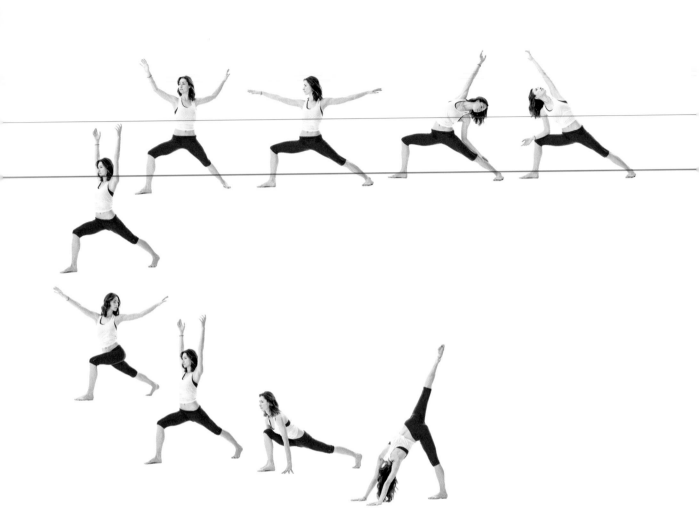

Take a big inhale and lift your right leg up and back to down dog split. Open up your hips if that feels nice for you. Exhale and step your foot through to low lunge. Press down through your legs and inhale up to high lunge. Exhale and twist to your left side and let your arms open wide. Inhale back to high lunge and open to warrior 2, spinning your back heel down so your toes point toward your front leg, and sink your hips. Bend your front knee over your front foot and open your arms out to your sides. Relax your head and neck and shoulders. Breathe here for a few moments. Let the inhales lift you up a bit and the exhales soften you a bit more.

Take a big inhale and tip your torso back to reverse warrior, sliding your back hand gently down your back leg and lift your opposite arm up. Tip forward into extended side angle, pressing your top forearm on your thigh and your opposite arm overhead. Roll your torso open if you'd like. Press your fingertips to the ground on either side of your front foot, take a big inhale, lift your hips up, and

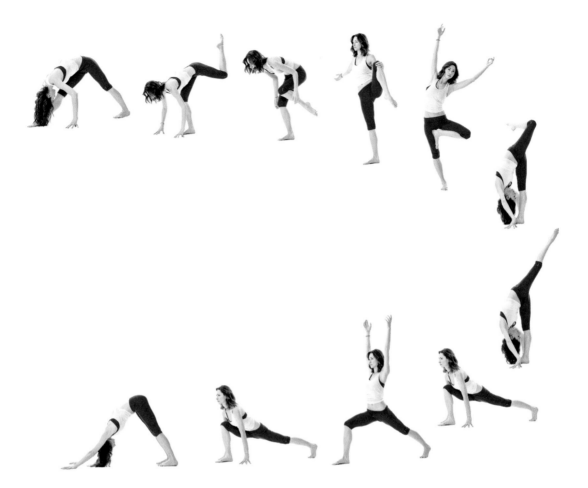

relax your torso over your front leg to single leg forward bend. Soften your knees, crawl your fingertips out in front of you, and let your back leg float up off the ground into warrior 3. Soften your knees and round up to stand, bringing your left shin in front of you for a squeeze for shin hug. Open your leg out to the side and press your foot into your thigh for tree. Open your arms overhead. Sway a bit here in the breeze if that feels nice.

When you are ready, give your shin another squeeze, inhale, and lift everything up. Exhale and dive your torso up and over for standing split. Press your fingertips on the ground for balance, relax your head and neck, and open your left leg behind you. Soften your knees and step your left foot back to low lunge. Press down through your legs and lift up to high lunge. Exhale back to low lunge and make your way back to down dog.

Repeat the movement phrase on the left side. Stay easy with your breath.

FORGET THE POSE

When you really start to feel the flow of your body moving with your breath, you'll feel one movement blending into the next with the calmness of a gentle stream. Allow the movements to really feel good for you. Feeling is the most important task here. The movements will become more natural and easy with practice, but they are not the goal. Sensitizing you to how you feel is the goal. Tapping into your intuition, restorative healing space, and expanding your physical capabilities all charge up simultaneously when you prioritize feeling. Forget the pose.

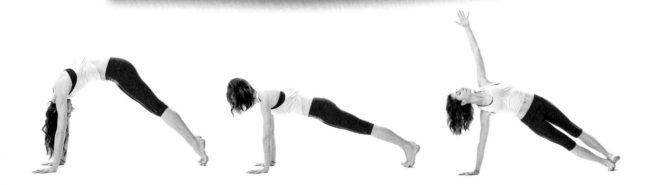

From down dog, sway a bit here to keep everything easy and soft. Tuck your chin and round out into plank, leading with your upper back like a wave. Shift your weight onto your right hand and the outside edge of your right foot. Take a big inhale, and open your torso toward your left for side plank. If you want some more

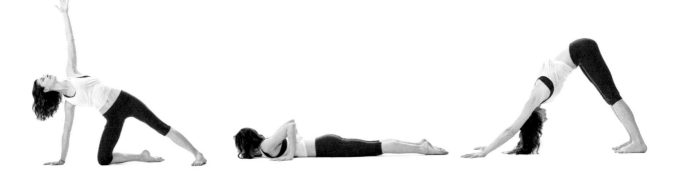

stability, soften your right shin to the ground for support. When you're ready, come back to plank and go for the other side. When you're ready, come back to plank. Soften your elbows and lower down to your belly. Take a big inhale and lift yourself up and back to down dog.

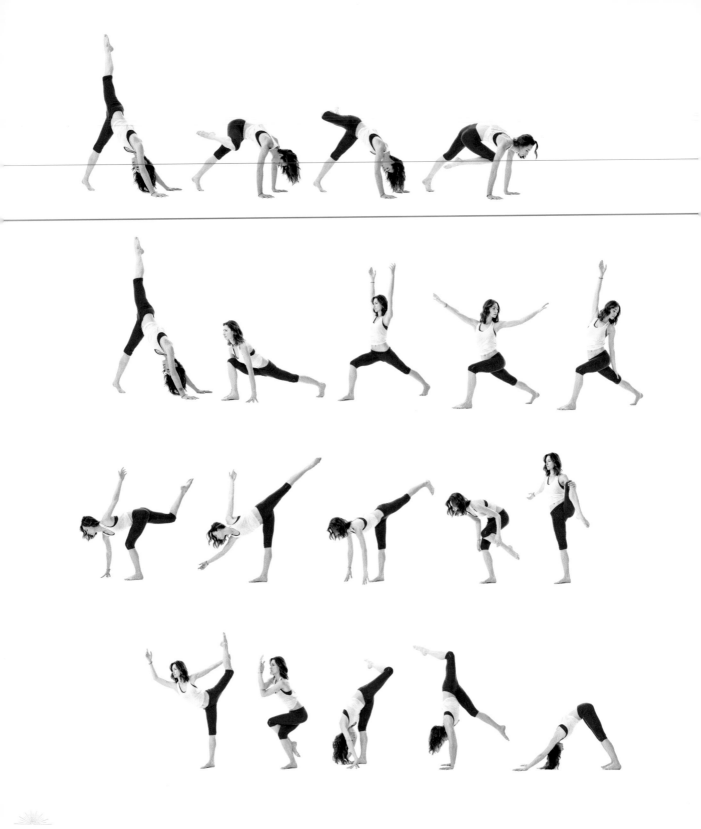

Take a big inhale and lift your right leg up and back to down dog split. Open your hips if that feels nice. Keeping your hips high, arc your right knee high and around to your right upper arm. Look forward and lean forward. Take a big inhale and lift your leg back to down dog split. Arc your knee across your body to your left upper arm. Look forward and lean forward. Take a big inhale back to down dog split. Exhale and step your foot through to low lunge. Inhale up to high lunge. Exhale and twist to your left side and let your arms open wide. Take a big inhale and tip back to reverse the twist. Tip forward to twisted half-moon, bringing your right fingertips to the ground as you tip forward. Soften your knees and shift your hips forward as you exhale. Let your back leg follow your hips and lift up. Open your left arm up and gaze up toward your top hand if you'd like. Stay easy and soft in your knees and shoulders as you twist. Press your right fingertips to the ground for support, exhale, and soften your knees through the center as you change sides. Take a big inhale and roll your body open to your left, opening your hips, belly, and shoulders. Lift your left arm up and gaze upward if that feels nice. Exhale as you soften your knees and bring your left fingertips to the ground, so both hands' fingertips are on the ground for support and your back leg is extended behind you.

Soften your knees and round up to stand, bringing your left shin in front of you and give it a squeeze. Roll around your hips here, keeping your standing leg soft in your knee. Drop your knee toward the ground and catch ahold of your shin with your left hand. Exhale and soften here. Take a big inhale and press your left shin into your left hand and lift your right arm up for your dancer pose. Exhale and soften your knees, let go of your left foot, and wrap your left leg in front and around your right leg in front of you, sinking through your hips. Wrap your left arm under your right arm and lift up through your fingertips for eagle. Unravel your legs and arms and dive up and over your standing leg, bringing your fingertips to the ground for support, and open your left leg and hips behind you for standing split. Drop your head and neck and roll around from your hips and belly to open up if that feels good. Plant your palms on the ground a couple of feet in front of your front foot. Inhale and rock forward a bit, shifting the weight onto your hands. Exhale and rock back. When you inhale and rock forward, move from your hips and belly, lifting your hips over your shoulders. Exhale, rock back, and relax. If this brings you into a little handstand hang time, play around, but keep it easy and enjoy! When you're ready, head back to down dog and settle here for a few long, deep breaths.

Repeat the movement phrase on your left side.

CREATE SPACE BY SOFTENING

When we have space in our bodies and minds, we feel great, connected, and joyful. When we are cramped, tight, and tense in our bodies and minds, we feel stuck, disconnected, and frustrated. The practice of softening as you move your body from one movement to the next is practical in the way of efficient, graceful movement. It also creates that expansive, amazing feeling of body and mind. The feeling is what we're going for. It's the basis of the practice and where all the good stuff rests. Softening is a big secret when it comes to the practice. You'll find relaxation, ease, peace, and calm from moment to moment when you simply let yourself soften and enjoy! Your inhale is the moment to expand, lift, and enjoy. Your exhale is the moment to soften, settle, or move easily. We can fully enjoy our expansive inhales when we allow ourselves to gracefully soften as we exhale. It all fits together like a wave, a song, and a dance. Enjoy the flow you create. The more you practice and experience flow on the mat, the more you just might start to notice a sweet kind of flow in your life.

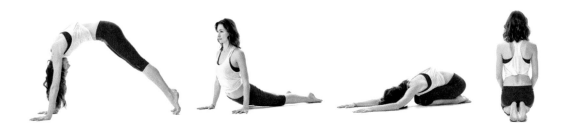

From down dog, tuck your chin and roll out to plank. Soften your knees to the ground and sink your hips toward the ground, letting your body roll side to side if that feels good. If this isn't so nice on your lower back, soften your elbows more and ease your torso closer toward the floor so you're opening up your middle and upper back. Soften your elbows and lower down to your belly. Press down through your palms and shift your hips back to child's pose. Rest here for a few moments. When you're ready, bring yourself up to sit on your heels. Close your eyes for a moment and draw your attention inward.

COME BACK
TO YOUR BREATH

Your entire flow is a moving meditation. The inhales lift and expand your body and invigorate your mind. The exhales move you a little farther physically and a little deeper inwardly. If you notice your mind wandering or thinking, that's natural. When you notice, draw your attention back inward, back to your breath. This practice of noticing and then coming back to your breath is a simple way to come back to the moment. If you feel yourself losing your breath, or getting frazzled with the movements, give yourself a moment to be still. Resting in child's pose and then coming up and sitting hips to heels or easy cross-legged is a nice place to reconnect during your practice. Don't feel pressured to accomplish movements. Make it your priority to come back to your breath. When you're with your breath, you're in the flow of becoming sensitized to how you feel. That's the awesome zone where all the good stuff happens.

❀

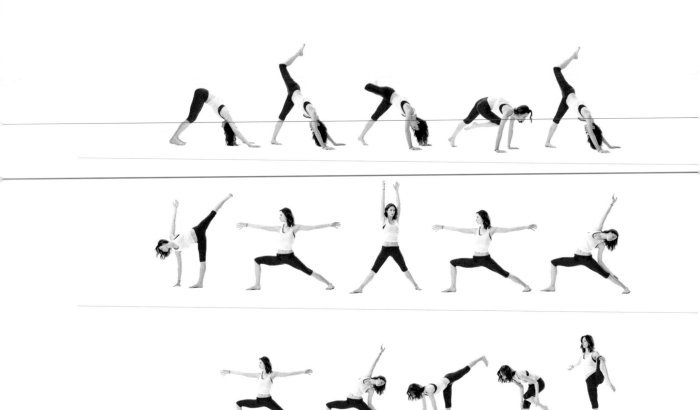

Come onto all fours, spread your fingers wide, take a big inhale, and lift your hips up and back to down dog. Soften here for a moment. Take a big inhale and lift your right leg up and back to down dog split. Open your hips if that feels nice. Keeping your hips high, arc your right knee high and around to your right upper arm. Look forward and lean forward. Take a big inhale and lift your leg back to down dog split. Arc your knee across your body to your left upper arm. Look forward and lean forward. Take a big inhale back to down dog split. Exhale and step your foot through to low lunge. Inhale up to high lunge. Exhale and twist to your left side and let your arms open wide. Take a big inhale and tip back to reverse the twist. Tip forward to your twisted half-moon, bringing your right fingertips to the ground as you tip forward. Soften your knees and shift your hips forward as you exhale. Let your back leg follow your hips and lift up. Open your left arm up and gaze up toward your top hand if you'd like. Stay easy and soft in your knees and shoulders as you twist. Press your left fingertips to the ground for support, exhale, and soften your knees through the center as you trade sides. Take a big inhale and roll your body open to your left, opening your hips, belly, and shoulders. Lift your right arm up and gaze upward if that feels nice.

Soften your knees and elbows and step your left leg back a few feet behind you. Press down through your legs, take a big inhale, and lift your hips and arms up. Exhale into warrior 2, bending your front knee over your front foot and opening your arms out to your sides. Turn your back toes (and foot) slightly in so you are getting a nice hip opener here. Take a big inhale and tip your torso back to reverse warrior, sliding your left hand gently down your back leg and lifting your right arm up. Lengthen your front leg by lifting your

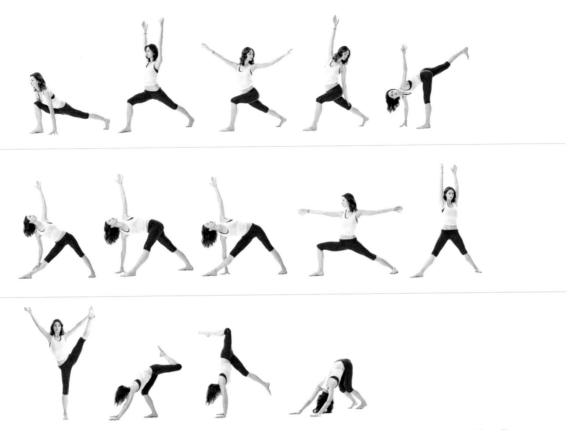

hips a bit. Tip forward to triangle sliding your right hand down your leg and landing on your shin or pressing your fingertips to the ground for support. Whatever feels nice. Open your left arm up and gaze upward if you want to. Soften your knees as you exhale. Press your right fingertips to the ground, twist toward your left, and open your left arm upward for twisted triangle. Gaze upward if that feels nice. Bringing it back around to triangle, soften your knees, press your right fingertips to the ground, roll your body open toward your left, and open your left arm upward. Gaze upward if that feels nice.

Soften your knees, reach your left arm behind you, press down through your legs, and take a big inhale and lift your hips and arms up. Exhale and soften back to warrior 2. Take a big inhale and lift your hips and arms up overhead. Exhale and settle back to warrior 2. Take a big inhale and tip back to reverse warrior, sliding your left hand gently down your back leg and lifting your right arm upward. Exhale and sweep forward, crawling your fingertips on the ground in front of you; bringing your torso forward, lift your left leg behind you for warrior 3. Soften your knees and round up to stand, bringing your left shin in front of you for a squeeze. Open your hips here if you'd like. Grab your heel, take a big inhale, and open your left leg out to your side a bit if that feels nice. Open your right arm out to your right for balance. Exhale and dive up and over your standing leg and press your palms on the ground a few feet in front of your front foot. Inhale and rock forward and back for your handstand rocks. When you're ready, find your way gently back to down dog.

Repeat on your other side.

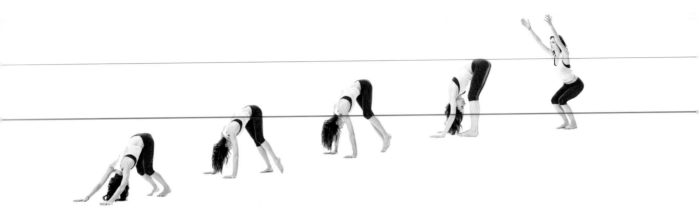

From down dog take an easy stroll to the top of your mat, coming into a standing forward bend. Soften your knees here as you hang your torso over your legs. Sink your hips, and take a big inhale to lift your torso and arms up into chair. Exhale, bring your palms together, and twist toward your left side, pressing your right elbow outside your left knee. Take a big inhale and come back to chair and twist to the other side. Take a big inhale and come back to chair. Exhale, interlace your hands behind you, and fold your torso over your legs. Relax your head and neck here and sway a bit to open up if that feels good. Release your hands to the ground for support, and sink your hips, coming into a squat. Bring your hands behind you on the ground for support and gently come to sit on your hips.

Lift your legs in front of you with your knees soft for boat. If this is too much on your lower back, press your hands or rest your forearms on the ground behind you for support. Lower your body halfway down toward the ground and lift back up, keeping your head, neck, and shoulders relaxed. Repeat this about 10 times with your breath. Lower halfway down and on your right side with your arms to the left for boat twist. Lift back up. Try on the left side and roll through this about 10 times with your breath. Lower down and open your arms behind you, pressing your lower back toward the ground. Take a big inhale here to open up. Exhale and hug your knees, relaxing on your back. Rock a bit side to side if that feels good. Rock gently forward and back to come up to stand. Press your hands on the ground in front of you and lift up into a standing forward bend, keeping your knees soft. Relax your head and neck here. Round up to stand one notch at a time. Take a big inhale and float your arms out and up overhead. Exhale and soften back into your standing forward bend. Press your palms on the ground and make your way gently back to down dog.

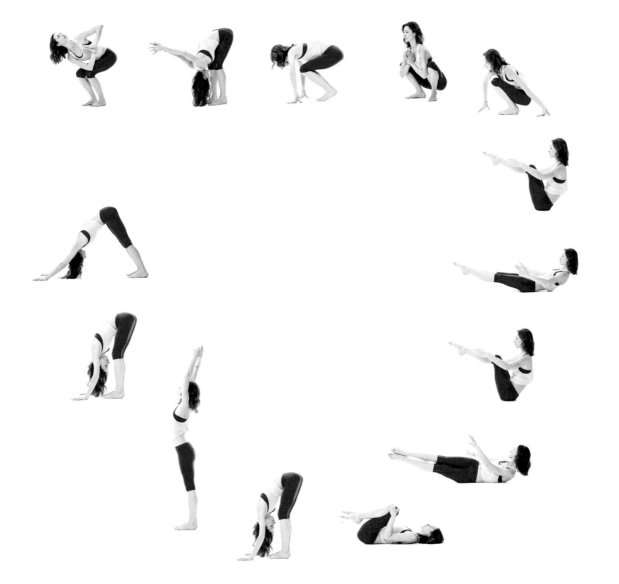

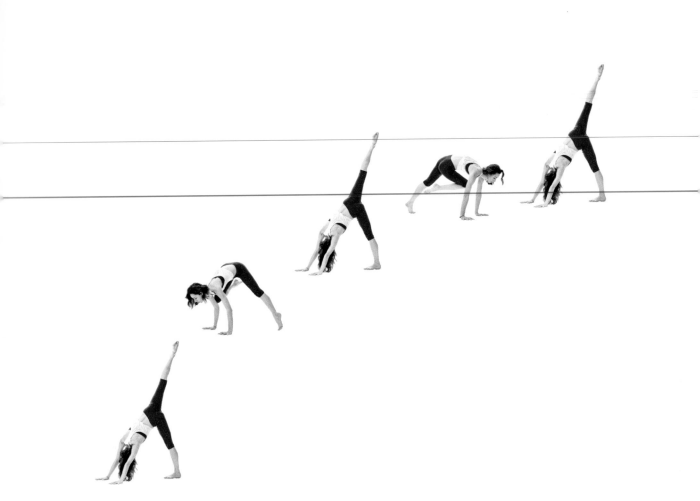

Take a big inhale and lift your right leg up and back to down dog split. Open your hips if that feels nice. Keeping your hips high, arc your right knee high and around to your right upper arm. Look forward and lean forward. Take a big inhale and lift your leg back to down dog split. Arc your knee across your body to your left upper arm. Look forward and lean forward. Take a big inhale back to down dog split. Exhale and step your foot through to low lunge. Ground your back heel down so your foot is placed on the ground, press down through your legs, and lift up into warrior 1, reaching your arms up overhead. Roll around in your hips and belly to find a nice place. Relax your arms down and interlace your hands behind you. Take a big inhale and lift your torso up. Exhale and relax your torso forward inside your front leg. Relax your head and neck.

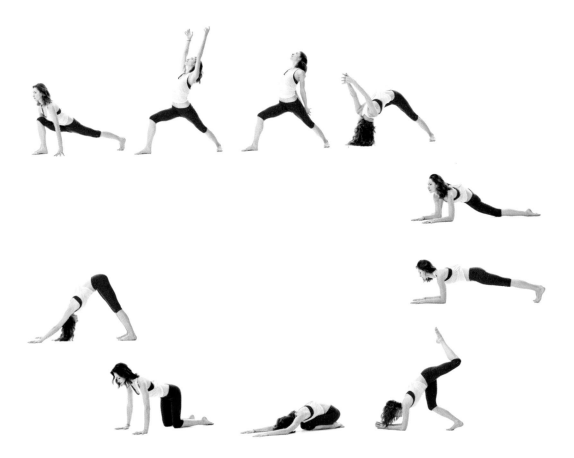

When you're ready, release your clasp and press your hands on the ground for support. Move your front foot out to your right a bit to make room for your hips. Soften your back knee to the ground and either stay here with straighter arms, or soften your elbows and come down to your forearms, however feels best for you. Hang here for a few long, deep breaths. When you're ready, come onto your forearms, lean to your left and slide your front leg behind you into forearm plank. Either stay here or walk your feet up toward your head. Take a big inhale and lift one leg up, rolling in your hips and belly. Exhale and soften the leg down and try on the other side. Roll through this a few times with your breath. If you have some hang time in forearm stand, that's fun, but keep it easy in your body and mind. Rest in child's pose for a few moments. When you're ready, come onto all fours, tuck your toes, and take a big inhale to lift your hips up and back to down dog.

HANDSTAND & FOREARM SECRET TIPS

Going upside down can cause all sorts of emotions to flood in suddenly. Everything from fear, to joy, to fun, to frustration could emerge. It's useful to practice the process of challenging movements not to achieve the movement, but to improve how we approach challenges. When we approach with ease, we not only accomplish more with less effort, but get in that flow state of relaxation and calm no matter what the circumstance. It's important to continue moving softly, from your hips and belly, as you practice the process of handstands and forearm stands. When you move from your hips, you are moving from the middle of your body and essentially letting the movement move you, instead of having to do a big haul to get yourself there. The movement of rolling around in your shin hug is the same as rolling around in your handstand and forearm stand rocks. Shin hug is a hip opener while standing on one leg. Handstand and forearm stand are hip openers while rocking off of one leg. Try rocking back and forth from shin hug to handstand to experience the easygoing movement and enjoyment of feeling handstand as a hip opener instead of a potentially scary movement. Same goes for forearm stand as you rock forward and back, moving from your hips and belly. Stay with your breath and enjoy.

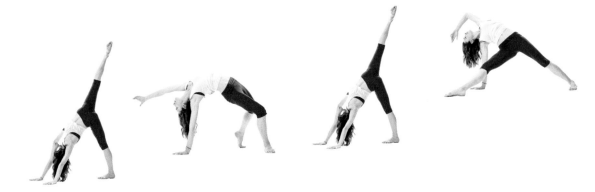

From down dog, take a big inhale and lift your right leg up and back to down dog split. Open your hips and shoulders so much that you tip over to rock star if that feels nice. Open your hips and belly upward. Soften your knees and bring yourself back around to down dog split. Slide your right foot through and outside your left hand on the ground. Open your left arm and belly upward to fallen triangle. Soften here and slide your right leg back to down dog split. Softly bring your shin to the

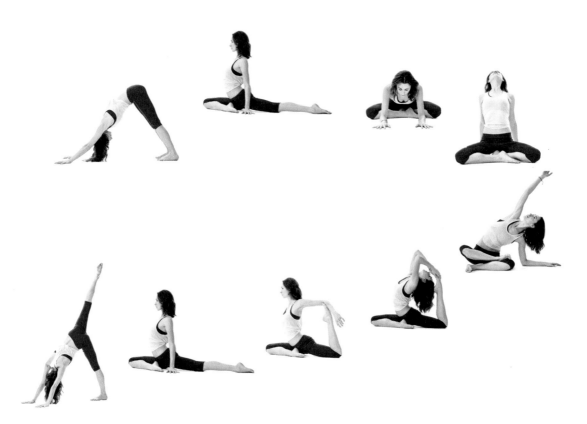

ground close to your hands to land in pigeon. Take a few moments to find a place where you feel a good opening and experience no pain. Either stay here, keeping your torso upright, or relax your torso forward. Hang here for several breaths to open. When you're ready, bring your torso back upright. If it feels good, bend your back knee and grab ahold of your ankle with your left hand to open up here.

Unwind out of that, shift your weight to your right hip, bring your back leg around, and stack your ankles and knees on top of each other. If that doesn't feel nice to you, rest your left shin in front of your right to sit easy, cross-legged, ankle to knee. Press your fingertips behind you on the ground for support; take a big inhale to lean back and open up here. Either stay here or walk your body forward or side to side if that feels nice. Hang here for several long, deep breaths. When you're ready, bring your torso back up; slide your top leg behind you and back to pigeon. Plant your palms on the ground and make your way back to down dog however that feels nice for you. Maybe lift your left leg up and open your hips a bit, or simply head back to down dog and shift your weight around a bit here to even out this side. Take a few breaths to soften here.

Go for the other side.

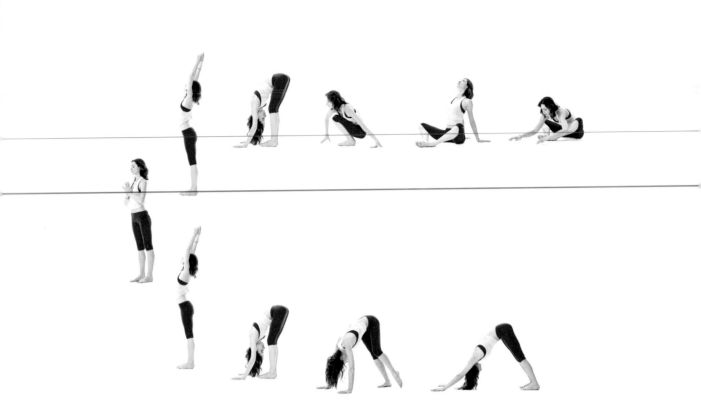

From down dog take an easy stroll up to the top of your mat to your standing forward bend. Relax your head and neck here and sway a bit if that feels nice to you. Roll up to stand one notch at a time. When you make it up, float your arms out and up. Press your palms together, close your eyes, and bring your thumbs to your heartbeat. Soften here for a moment. Soften your knees. Relax your head and neck and shoulders. Sway a bit side to side. Take a big inhale and lift your arms up. Exhale and soften over your legs. Press your palms on the ground, shift some weight into your arms, and come to an easy squat. Open up here, rolling your torso side to side if that feels nice. When you're ready, bring your hands behind you for support and come to sit.

Bring the bottoms of your feet together and let your knees open out to your sides. Press your hands behind you on the ground for support. Take a big inhale, lean back, and open up here. Either stay here if this feels nice, or crawl your torso forward to relax. Hang here for several deep breaths. Roll yourself down to lie on your back. Bring your knees along with you for the ride to be easy on your back. Either stay here and rock a bit side to side if that feels good or roll your torso up and over so your feet come toward the ground for plow. If plow doesn't feel nice on your neck and back, roll on down and relax. If you feel great in your plow, either stay here or press your palms to support your back and lift your legs up to shoulder stand. Hang here for several long, deep breaths.

When you are ready, soften your knees back around your ears and gently roll down to lie on your back. If you'd like to open up your back a bit more, try for bridge. Press

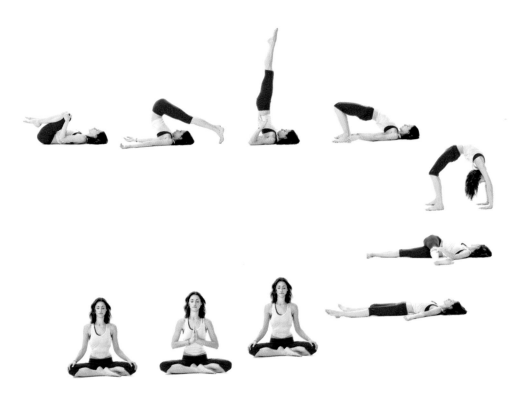

the bottoms of your feet on the ground under your hips. Relax your arms down by your sides. Gently press down through your feet and arms to lift up to bridge. Stay here for a few deep breaths and gently lower down. For wheel, press your palms on the ground next to your ears. Press down through your feet and hands to lift up into wheel. Hang here for a few deep breaths and gently lower down to the ground. If you'd like to take a gentle twist, let your leg drift to one side and rest for a few deep breaths. Open your arms out to the side to relax. Try the same on the other side. When you are ready to relax, stretch out a bit, close your eyes, and rest for several breaths.

When you're ready to come out of this, invite some more air back in. Roll around your wrists and ankles if that feels nice. Make your way up to sit easily and comfortably. Take your time. Come to a simple, easy seat. Close your eyes and draw your attention back inward. Take a big inhale and float your arms out and up. Press your palms together and bring your thumbs to your heartbeat. Soften here for a moment. Take a big inhale through your nose. Long exhale through your mouth. Twice more like that, big inhale, long exhale. One more time, big inhale, long exhale. When you are ready, relax your hands on your thighs and gently open your eyes.

You did it! Great job. I hope you feel energized, relaxed, and open.

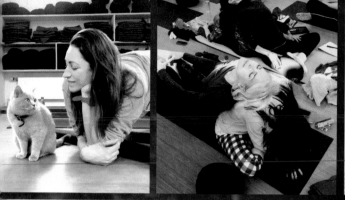
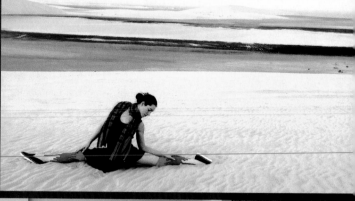
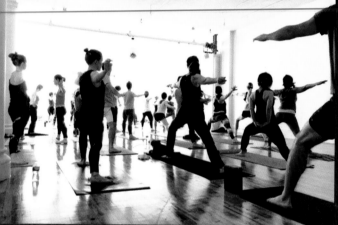
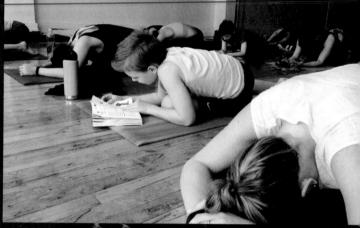
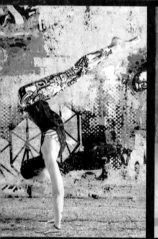
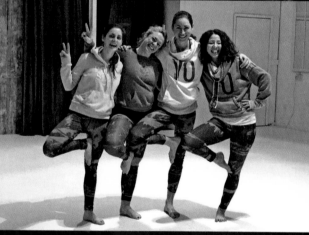
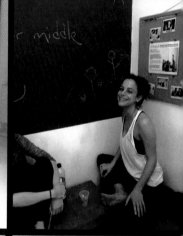
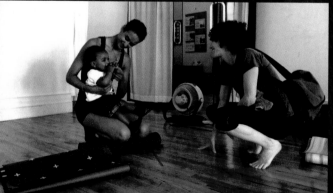
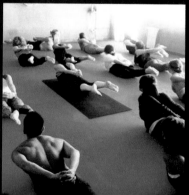
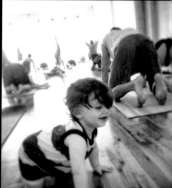

CHAPTER 7

RELAX

This practice is designed to de-stress your whole self, dissolving tension as you move easily through the flow. Enjoy!

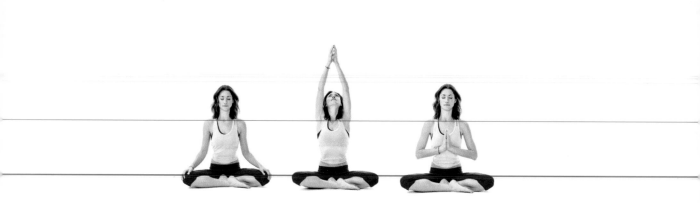

Start sitting however you can be comfortable. Close your eyes and rest your attention on your breath. If you notice your attention shifting, see if you can guide it right back to your breath.

Take a big inhale and lift your arms up overhead. Close your eyes, bring your palms together, and bring your thumbs to your heartbeat. Soften here for a moment. Take a big inhale through your nose. Long exhale out through your mouth. Twice more like that. Big inhale, long exhale. One more time, big inhale and long exhale. When you are ready, gently relax your hands back on your thighs and open your eyes.

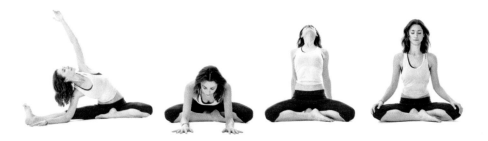

Staying easy in your body, open your right leg out to your side, lean to your right, resting your right hand and forearm on the ground on your side. Open your left arm up and over your head. Hang here for a few breaths, moving your body gently to open things up a bit. When you're ready, come back up to the middle and go for the other side. When you're ready, bring your legs back to a comfortable, easy seated position. Walk your hands forward and let your torso relax. Sway a bit here if that feels nice for you. When you are ready, gently bring yourself back up to the middle. Press your fingertips behind you on the ground, take a big inhale, and lift your chest and hips up. As you exhale, relax to your middle. Rest your hands on your thighs and close your eyes for a moment, guiding your attention back to your breath.

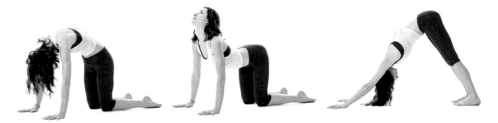

Staying soft and easy in your body, come onto all fours. Start to move a bit with your breath, moving your torso side to side, round and round, and forward and back, however feels good for you. When you're ready, tuck your toes, take a big inhale, and lift your hips up and back to down dog. Move around a bit here how it feels good for you to get comfortable and open up a bit.

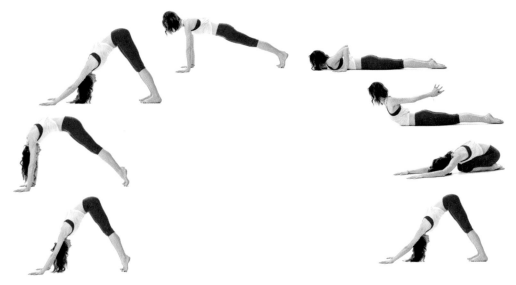

Take a big inhale and lift up on your tippy toes. Exhale and relax back. Twice more just like that, big inhale and lift, easy exhale and soften. One more time, big inhale and lift, easy exhale and soften. Tuck your chin and roll out into a plank pose. Sway around here a bit if that feels nice. Take a big inhale and lift your hips up and back to down dog. Once more just like that, tuck your chin and round on out into plank. This time, soften your elbows and lower down to your belly. Interlace your hands behind you and lift up a bit, swaying side to side, however feels good for you. When you're ready, soften back to your belly. Press your palms on the ground under your shoulders. Keeping your knees on the ground, shift your hips back to child's pose. Rest here for a moment. When you're ready, lift your hips, tuck your toes, and lift up and back into down dog.

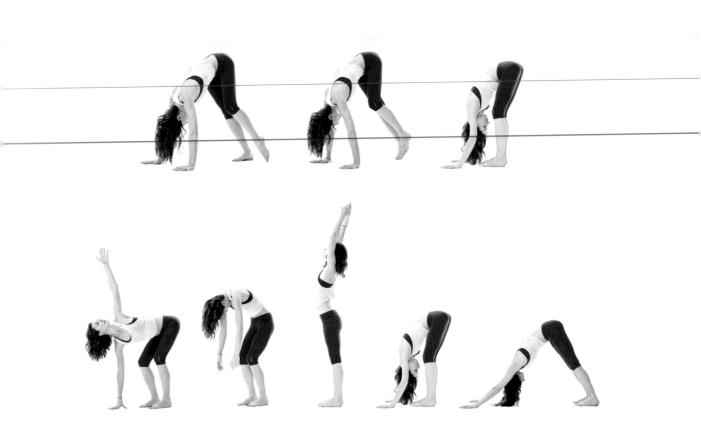

Take an easy walk up to your hands. Let your hands move to free up some space if you'd like. Come into your easy standing forward bend. Soften your knees to make some space for your hamstrings if that feels good. Relax your head and neck and breathe here for a bit. Soften your knees, press your right fingertips on the ground, take a big inhale, and open your body to your left, extending your left arm up. Gaze up if you want to. Exhale and come through the middle and go for the other side, pressing your left fingertips on the ground and opening your body to the right, extending your right arm up. Gaze up if that feels nice. When you're ready, exhale and come to center. Keeping your head and neck soft, roll up to stand one notch at a time. When you make it up, take a big inhale and float your arms out and up. Easy exhale and round back into standing forward bend. Go for that twice more with your breath rounding up and down softly. Plant your palms and find your way back to down dog, stepping or moving however it feels great to you.

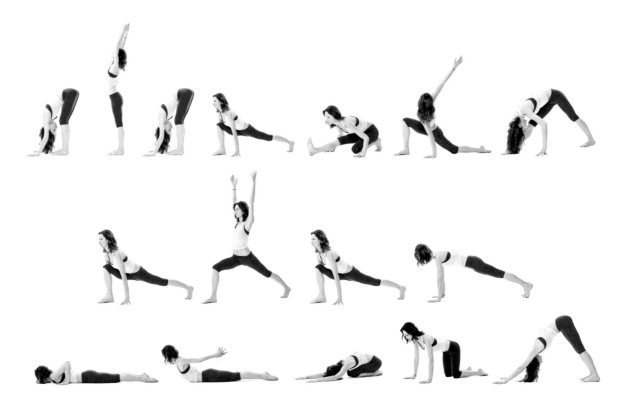

From down dog, take an easy stroll to the top of your mat. Hang easy in standing forward bend. Roll up to stand one notch at a time. Once you are up, take a big inhale and float your arms out and up. Exhale and soften back to your forward bend. Soften your knees, press your fingertips on the ground, and step your left leg back into low lunge. Sink your hips and move here to open up a bit. Ease your back knee to the ground. If it feels nice, keep your torso relaxed forward or open yourself upward, lifting your arms if that feels better. Explore here for a bit to open up.

When you're ready, press your fingertips on the ground on either side of your front foot; keeping your back knee on the ground, shift your hips toward your back heel. Relax your torso over your extended leg. Relax your head and neck. Crawl yourself back to your low lunge, press your left fingertips to the ground, take a big inhale, and open your right arm and torso toward your right. As you exhale, press both fingertips to the ground on either side of your front foot. Take a big inhale and lift your hips up as you relax your torso over your front leg. Sway a bit here if that feels nice. Sink your hips, coming back into your low lunge. Take a big inhale and lift up to high lunge. Exhale to low lunge, plant your palms on the ground, and step back to plank. Soften your elbows and lower down to your belly. Interlace your hands behind you, take a big inhale, and lift up gently. When you're ready, soften back to the ground. Press your palms on the ground and shift back to child's pose. When you're ready, come back to all fours, spread your fingers wide, tuck your toes, take a big inhale, and lift your hips up and back to down dog.

Repeat the movement phrase on the other side.

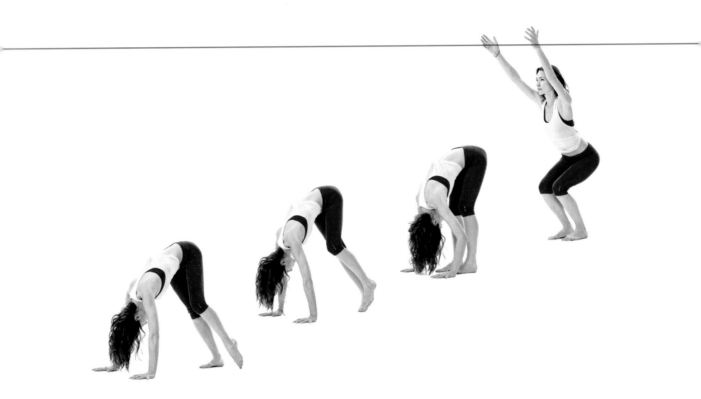

Walk your feet up to the top of your mat and come into an easy standing forward bend. Let your head and neck relax here for a few breaths. Sink your hips, take a big inhale, and lift your torso and arms up into chair. Press your thumbs to your heartbeat and twist toward your left, bringing your right elbow outside your left knee. Take a big inhale, lift back into chair, and take

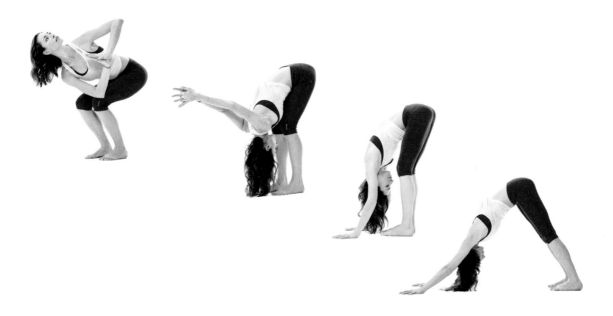

an easy twist to your other side. Take a big inhale and lift back into chair. Exhale and fold over your legs, interlacing your hands behind you, and relax your head, neck, and shoulders. Hang here for a few breaths. When you're ready, release your hands and come back into standing forward bend. Press your palms to the ground and make your way back to down dog.

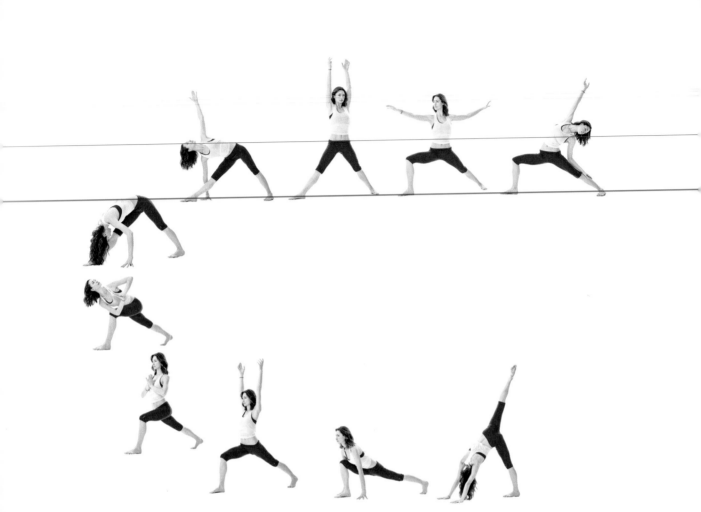

Take a big inhale and lift your right leg up to down dog split. Open your hips and shoulders if that feels nice. Exhale and step your foot through to low lunge. Take a big inhale and lift up to high lunge. Bring your palms together and soften them into your heartbeat. Take a big inhale to lift up, and exhale, twisting to your left side, bringing your right elbow outside your left knee. When you're ready, bring both fingertips to the ground on either side of your front foot and lift your hips up and relax your torso over your legs for your single leg forward bend. Sway a bit side to side. Ground your back heel down, spin your torso toward your left, and open into triangle. Lift your left arm up and gaze up if that feels nice for you. Soften your knees, reach your top arm back, press down through your legs, and lift your hips and arms up for warrior 2 lift. Soften your hips; bending your front knee over your front foot, relax your arms out to the sides for warrior 2. Tip your torso back, sliding your left hand gently down your back leg, lifting your right arm up for reverse warrior.

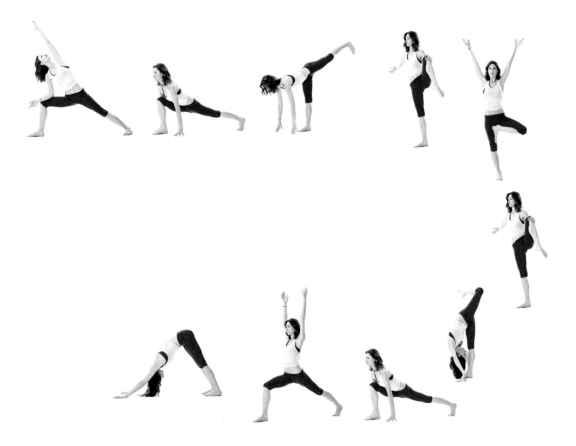

Tip your torso forward, pressing your right forearm on your right thigh and opening your left arm up and overhead for extended side angle. Roll your torso open if that feels good.

Bring your fingertips to the ground and come into a low lunge. Relax your head, neck, and shoulders and sway a bit here. When you're ready, soften your knees, crawl your fingertips out in front of you a bit, and let your back leg float up behind you into warrior 3. Soften your knees and round up to stand. Squeeze your left shin in front of you. Roll your hips around a bit here if that feels nice. Press the bottom of your left foot into your right inner thigh, or press your toes on the ground and let your heel rest on your right calf if that's easier for you. Open your arms upward for your tree. Hang here for a few long, deep breaths. Sway a bit side to side. Take a big inhale, hug your left shin back into your chest, and lift up here. As you exhale, dive up and over your standing leg bringing your fingertips to the ground for support for standing split. Relax your head and neck. Soften your knees and step your top leg back to low lunge. Press down through your legs, take a big inhale and lift up to high lunge. Exhale back down, plant your palms, and find your way back to down dog.

Repeat the movement phrase on the other side.

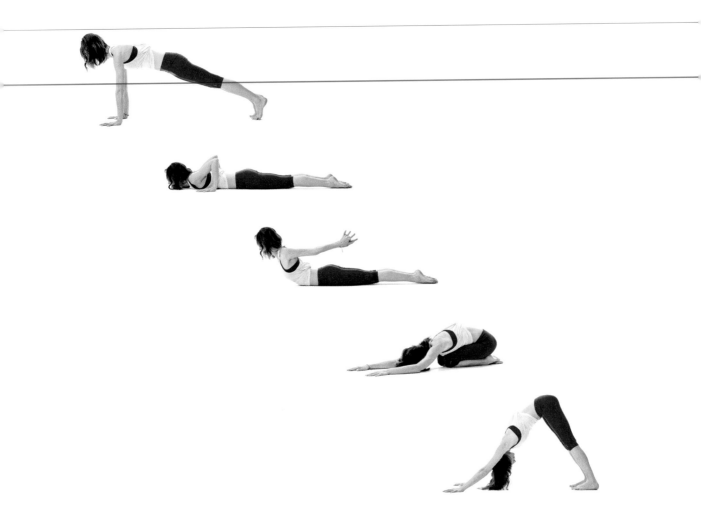

Round out to plank. Soften your elbows and lower down to your belly. Interlace your hands behind you, take a big inhale, and lift your torso up a bit. Sway side to side if that feels nice. When you are ready, soften your torso back to the ground. Press your palms on the ground and shift your hips back to your heels for child's pose. Rest here for a few breaths. When you're ready, press your palms into the ground, take a big inhale, and lift up and back to down dog.

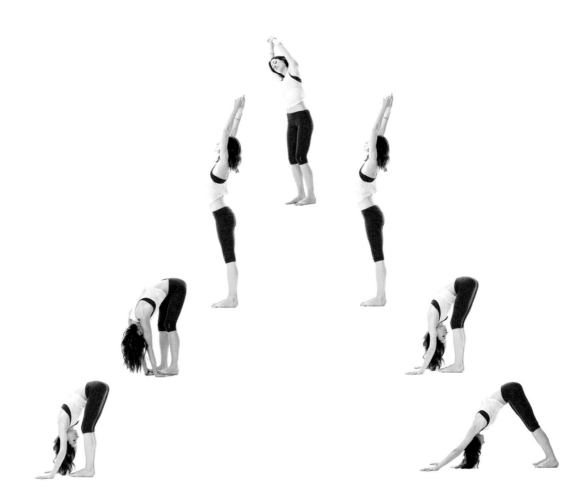

Walk your hands gently back to your feet so you're in a standing forward bend at the back of your mat. Step on your hands so the tops of your hands are on the ground and your fingers face toward your heels. Relax your head and neck. Soften your knees a bit and hang here for a few long, deep breaths. Release your hands and roll up to stand one notch at a time. When you make it up, take a big inhale and float your arms out and up. Grab hold of your left wrist with your right hand, lift up and over toward your right a bit, allowing your body to move how it feels good. When you're ready, come back to center and go for the other side. When you're ready, let go of the hold, take a big inhale, lifting your arms up, exhale, and relax your torso over your legs. Walk yourself gently back out to down dog.

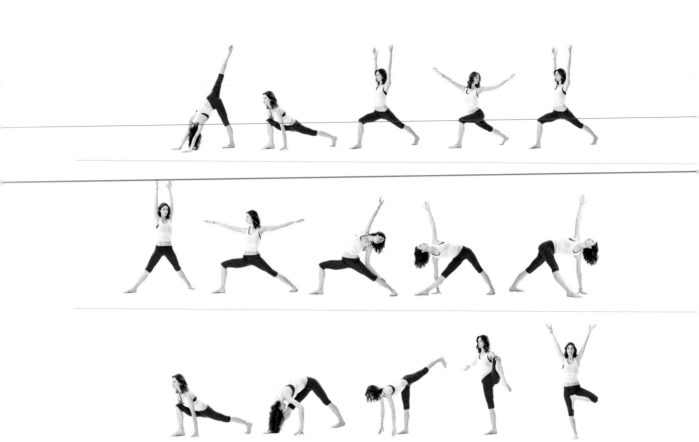

Take a big inhale and lift your right leg up and back to down dog split. Open your hips and shoulders if that feels nice. Step your foot forward to low lunge. Take a big inhale and lift up to high lunge. Exhale as you twist toward your left side and let your arms open wide. Inhale back to high lunge. Repeat that twice more. Exhale, twist toward your left, and let your arms open wide. Inhale back to high lunge. Exhale, twist toward your left, and let your arms open wide. Inhale back to high lunge and keep opening, rolling your back heel down to the ground to warrior 2. Open your arms out to your sides and relax your head, neck, and shoulders.

Take a big inhale as you lift your hips and arms up. Exhale and soften back to warrior 2. Inhale and tip back to reverse warrior, sliding your back hand gently down your back leg and arching your top arm up. Lengthen your front leg, leaning back a little farther. Tip your torso up and over to triangle, sliding your right hand down your leg, either resting on your shin or bringing your fingertips to the ground. Lift your left arm up and gaze up if that feels nice for you. Soften your knees, press your left fingertips to the ground, and roll your body open toward your right, opening your right arm up to twisted triangle. When you're ready, bring your right fingertips to the ground and open back to open triangle. Soften your knees, press down through your legs, take a big inhale, and lift back into warrior 2, lifting your hips and arms up. Exhale and soften back to warrior 2, opening your arms out to your sides.

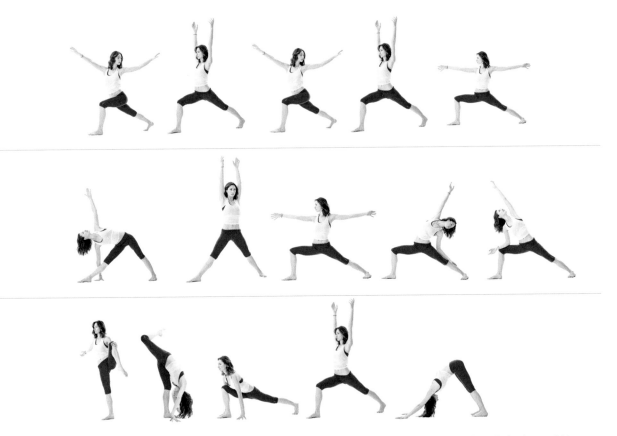

Take a big inhale and tip your torso back to your reverse warrior. Exhale and tip your torso forward to your extended side angle, pressing your top arm on your front thigh and your other arm up overhead. Roll your torso open if that feels nice. When you're ready, bring your fingertips to the ground and sink your hips to low lunge. Take a big inhale and lift your hips up to single leg forward bend, relaxing your torso over your front leg. Soften your knees, crawl your fingertips out in front of you, and let your back leg lift up to warrior 3. Soften your knees and round up to stand, bringing your left shin in front of you and giving it a gentle squeeze. Open your hips and press the bottom of your foot into your upper thigh, or rest your toes on the ground and the bottom of your foot on your calf if that is better for your balance. Lift your arms up and hang here for a few long, deep breaths. Let yourself sway a bit to stay easy in the balance.

Take a big inhale and hug your shin back in front of you. Dive up and over to standing split, bringing your fingertips to the ground for support. Relax your head and neck. Soften your knees and step back to low lunge. Press down through your legs and lift up to high lunge. Exhale and come back down, press your palms on the ground, and make your way back to down dog.

Repeat this movement phrase on the other side.

STRENGTH IN SOFTNESS

You have a lot of power when you move softly, so allow your body to soften as you move. Stay easy in your knees and elbows, and let yourself move from your hips and belly. Your power comes from the middle of your body and flows through you easily when your joints are soft. When you soften in your joints and move from your middle, you can accomplish so much more with a lot less effort. The effect is massive strength in softness. You don't need to tense, force, struggle, and grit your way through. If you do, you'll get much less out of your practice. All that grit stands in your way of achieving everything more easily.

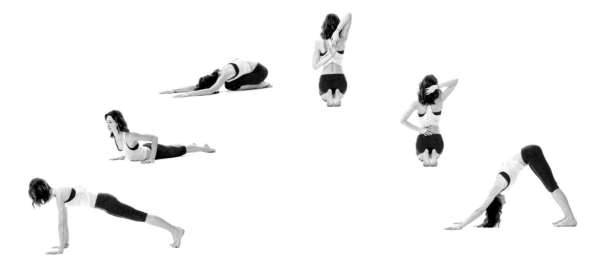

Roll out to plank. Soften your knees down to the ground, sink your hips, roll your shoulders down, take a big inhale, and open to up dog. Keeping your knees on the ground, relax your hips to your heels and come into child's pose. Rest here for a few breaths. When you're ready, come up to sit on your heels. Take a big inhale and float your arms up. Drop your left arm down and behind you. Bend your right elbow and bring your hands toward each other on your back. If your hands hook, join them together. If they don't hook, give yourself some space between them and soften. Hang here for a few long, deep breaths, moving a bit to open up if that feels nice. When you're ready, release your hands and go for the other side. Staying soft and easy, find your way back to down dog.

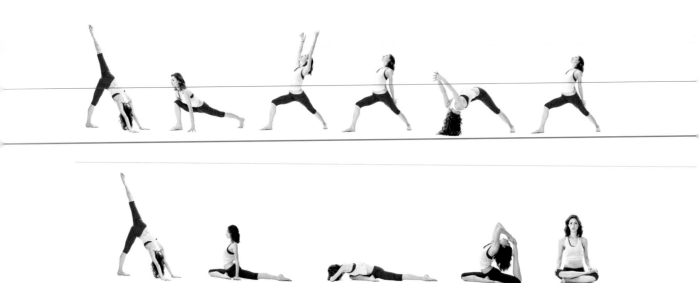

Take a big inhale and lift your right leg up and back to down dog split. Open your hips and shoulders if that feels nice. Exhale and step your foot through to low lunge. Ground your back heel down so your foot is on the ground, press down through your legs, and lift up into warrior 1, reaching your arms up overhead. Roll around in your hips and belly to find a nice place. When you're ready, relax your arms down and interlace your hands behind you. Take a big inhale and lift your torso up. Exhale and relax your torso forward inside your front leg. Relax your head and neck. When you're ready, press down through your legs, take a big inhale, and roll your torso up. Exhale and relax your torso forward inside your front leg again. When you're ready, release your clasp and press your hands on the ground for support. Move your front foot out to your right a bit to make room for your hips. Soften your back knee to the ground and either stay here with straighter arms, or soften your elbows and come down to your forearms, however feels best for you. Hang here for a few long, deep breaths.

If you feel good in your hips, feel free to hang here for a while. If you'd like to open your hamstrings a bit, shift your hips back toward your back heel, coming into your runner's stretch. Hang here for a few deep breaths. If this is enough of an opening, hang here. If it feels nice to slide your heel out in front of you for a split, go for that. Move slowly so you find a place where you feel a nice opening and can still breathe easily and fully. Hang here for a few long, deep breaths. When you're ready, slide your front foot back behind you to down dog split. Open your hips and shoulders if you'd like. Exhale and slide your front shin forward for pigeon.

Either stay upright with your torso if that feels nice, or crawl yourself forward, exploring around to one side and then the other. Find a nice place to rest for several long, deep breaths. When you're ready, bring your torso upright. Take an easy twist to your right side. If

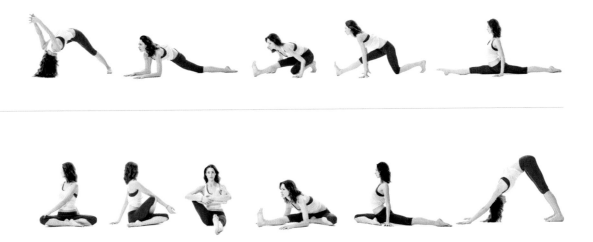

it feels good, open your torso gently toward your left side. If you can comfortably bend your back knee and draw your foot in for your full pigeon, go for it. If there is any tweaking in your body or it doesn't feel good, back off. When you're ready, unravel out of that one. Lean into your front hip and swing your back leg around for ankle to knee. If this doesn't feel nice in your joints, bring your left leg in front of your right leg for an easy comfortable seat. Either stay upright or bring your fingertips behind you; take a big inhale and lean back to open up. Stay here if you'd like, or if you'd like to crawl yourself forward over your legs, go for that. Maybe take a gentle walk with your hands around twisting to one side and an easy stroll around to the other side and find a nice place to relax for several long, deep breaths.

When you're ready, hug your right shin in toward you to open up your hips a bit. Slide your left leg out in front of you. Take a big inhale and give your right shin a squeeze. Exhale and place your foot on the ground outside your right leg. Take a big inhale and float your right arm up. Exhale and cross your arm over your leg, pressing your left fingertips on the ground behind you for support. Inhale and lift your torso up tall. Exhale and twist around a little farther. Repeat this a few times with your breath and then unwind toward the other side. When you're ready, bring your torso back to your center, and press your left foot on the ground so the bottom of your foot rests against your right thigh. Take a big inhale and lift up your torso a bit. Exhale and crawl yourself forward over your front leg. Soften your knee to make space for your hamstring if that feels nice. Hang here for several breaths. When you're ready, bring your torso back upright. Hug your left shin back in toward you. Bring your right leg back in, as well. Slide your left leg behind you back to pigeon. Plant your palms on the ground and make your way back to down dog.

Repeat this movement phrase on the other side.

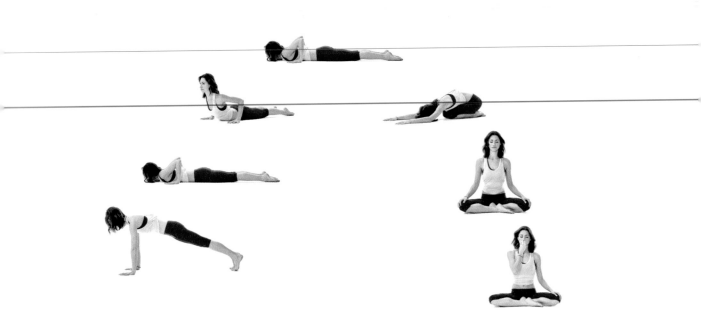

Roll out to plank. Soften your elbows and lower down to your belly. Press your palms on the ground next to your chest, take a big inhale, and lift up a bit. Hang here for a few breaths. When you're ready, soften back to relax on your belly. Press your palms on the ground and sink your hips to your heels, coming into child's pose. Rest here for a few breaths. When you're ready, come up to sit comfortably, cross-legged or hips to heels or another way that is comfortable for you.

From seated, relax your hands on your thighs, close your eyes, and bring your attention to your breath. With your right hand, make a peace sign. Curl your two top fingers in toward your palm so your pinkie, ring finger, and thumb are up. Relax your hand and press your ring finger onto your left nostril. Take a big inhale through your right nostril. Close off your right nostril with your thumb and hold the air for a moment. When you're ready, release your ring finger and let the air out of your left nostril. Take a big inhale through the left nostril, close off the left side with your ring finger, and hold the air for a moment. Release your thumb and let the air out of your right nostril. Continue alternating the breath for a few minutes. If you notice your attention drifting away from your breath, see if you can guide your attention back inward, right back to your breath. When you've had enough, relax your hands back on your thighs and gently open your eyes.

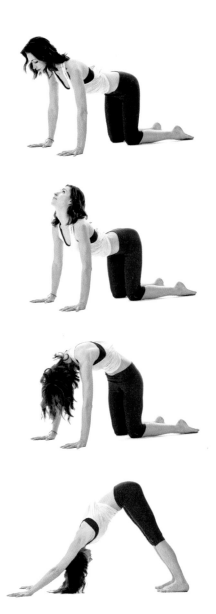

Staying soft and easy in your body, bring yourself to all fours. Roll around your torso however it feels good for you. Try inhaling as you drop your belly and look upward, and exhaling as you round your back and look inward. Feel free to move more freely to open up here. When you're ready, tuck your toes, take a big inhale, and lift your hips up and back to down dog.

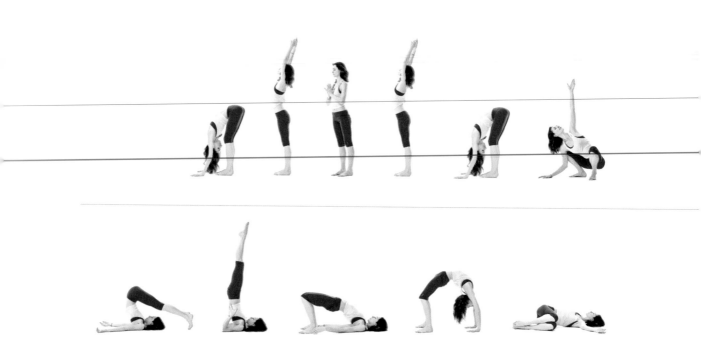

From down dog take an easy stroll up to the top of your mat to standing forward bend. Relax your head and neck here and sway a bit. Roll up to stand one notch at a time. When you make it up, float your arms out and up. Press your palms together, close your eyes, and bring your thumbs to your heartbeat. Soften here for a moment. Soften your knees. Relax your head, neck, and shoulders. Sway a bit side to side if that feels nice. Take a big inhale and lift your arms up. Exhale and soften over your legs. Press your palms on the ground, shift some weight into your arms, and come to an easy squat. Open up here, rolling your torso side to side if you'd like. When you're ready, bring your hands behind you for support and come to sit.

Bring the bottoms of your feet together and let your knees open out to your sides. Press your hands behind you on the ground for support. Take a big inhale, lean back, and open up here. Either stay here if this feels nice or crawl your torso forward to relax. Hang here for several deep breaths. When you're ready, roll yourself down to lie on your back. To be easy on your back, bring your knees along with you for the ride. Either stay here and rock a bit side to side if that feels nice, or roll your torso up and over so your feet come toward the ground for plow. If plow doesn't feel nice on your neck and back, roll on down and relax. If you feel great in your plow, either stay here or press your palms to support your back and lift your legs up to shoulder stand. Hang here for several long, deep breaths.

When you're ready, soften your knees back around your ears and gently roll down to lie on your back. If you'd like to open up your back a bit more, try for

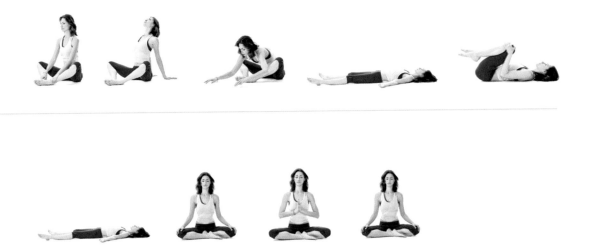

bridge. To do this, press the bottoms of your feet on the ground under your hips. Relax your arms down by your sides. Gently press down through your feet and arms to lift up. Stay here for a few deep breaths and gently lower down. For wheel, press your palms on the ground next to your ears. Press down through your feet and hands to lift up into wheel. Hang here for a few deep breaths and then gently lower down. If you'd like to take a gentle twist, let your knees drift to one side and rest for a few deep breaths. Open your arms out to the side to relax. Try the same on the other side. When you are ready to relax, stretch out a bit, close your eyes, and rest for several breaths.

When you're ready to come out of this, invite some more air back in. Roll around your wrists and ankles if that feels nice. Make your way up to sit easily and comfortably. Take your time. Come to a simple, easy seat. Close your eyes and draw your attention back inward. Take a big inhale and float your arms out and up. Press your palms together and bring your thumbs to your heartbeat. Soften here for a moment. Take a big inhale through your nose. Long exhale through your mouth. Twice more like that, big inhale, long exhale. One more time, big inhale, long exhale. When you are ready, relax your hands on your thighs and gently open your eyes.

I hope you feel relaxed and calm. Practice this routine anytime you would like to relax and de-stress.

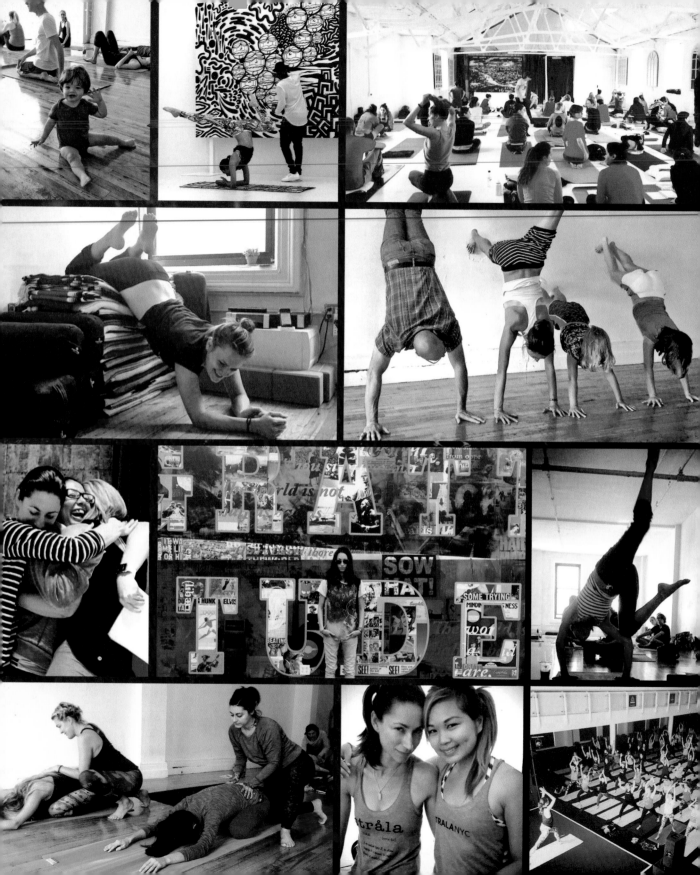

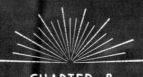

BASICS

This practice is designed to get you comfortable moving in your body in an easygoing way, while evenly building strength and a healthy range of motion, all the while resting your attention calmly on your breath. This routine is great if you are just getting started with your practice or if you feel like a simple routine to get back to basics. Breathe deeply and enjoy!

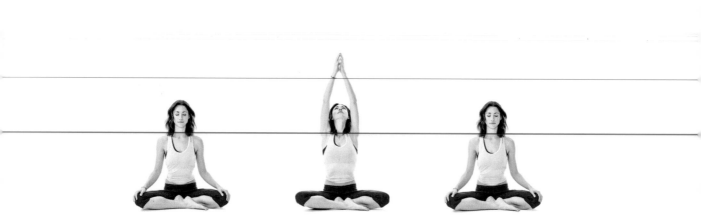

Start sitting, however you are comfortable. Close your eyes and rest your attention on your breath. If you notice your attention shifting, see if you can guide it back to your breath.

Take a big inhale and lift your arms up overhead. Close your eyes, bring your palms together, and bring your thumbs to your heartbeat. Soften here for a moment. Take a big inhale through your nose. Long exhale out through your mouth. Twice more like that. Big inhale, long exhale. One more time. Big inhale, long exhale. When you are ready, gently relax your hands on your thighs.

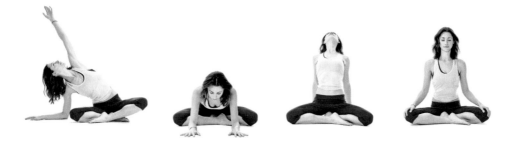

Staying soft, press your right hand on the ground to your side. Bend your torso to the side. Soften your elbow, resting your forearm on the ground and bring your left arm up high. Stay here for a few moments. Bring your torso up through the center and do the same on the other side. Walk your torso forward and relax your head and neck. Hang here for a few long, deep breaths. When you're ready, bring yourself back to center. Bring your hands behind you on the ground and lean back, lifting your chest and hips up if that feels good. When you're ready, come back to center.

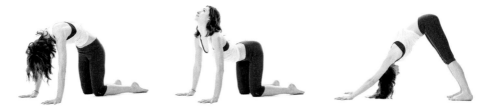

Staying soft and easy in your body, come onto all fours. Start to move a bit with your breath, moving your torso side to side, round and round, and forward and back, however feels good for you. Try inhaling as you drop your belly and look upward, and exhaling as you round your back and look inward. Feel free to move more freely to open up here. When you're ready, tuck your toes, take a big inhale, and lift your hips up and back to down dog. Move around a bit here to get comfortable and open up a bit.

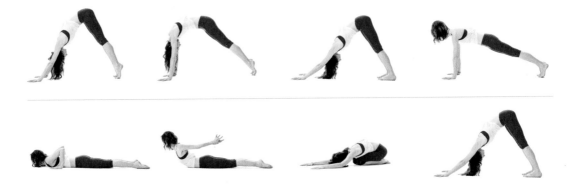

Take a big inhale and lift up on your tippy toes. Exhale and relax back. Twice more just like that, big inhale and lift, easy exhale and soften. One more time, big inhale and lift, easy exhale and soften. Tuck your chin and roll out into plank. Sway around here a bit if that feels nice. Take a big inhale and lift your hips up and back to down dog. Once more just like that, tuck your chin and round out into plank. This time, soften your elbows and lower down to your belly. Interlace your hands behind you and lift up a bit, swaying side to side, however feels good for you. When you're ready, soften back to your belly. Press your palms on the ground under your shoulders. Keep your knees on the ground and shift your hips back to child's pose. Rest here for a moment. When you're ready, lift your hips, tuck your toes, and lift up and back into down dog.

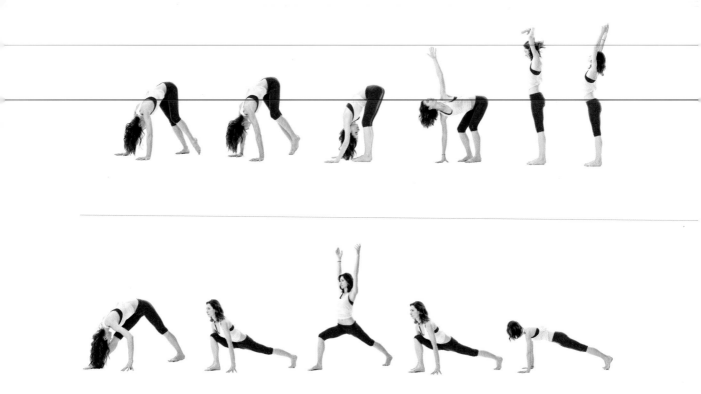

Walk your feet up to the top of your mat and come into a standing forward bend. Soften your knees and press your right fingertips to the ground. Open your body and left arm up toward your left. Gaze upward if that feels nice. When you're ready, come back to center and go for the other side. Keeping your head and neck soft, round up to stand one notch at a time. Once you make it up to stand, take a big inhale and float your arms out and up. Exhale and soften back to your standing forward bend.

Soften your knees, press your fingertips to the ground, and step your left leg back to low lunge. Sway a bit here. Soften your back knee to the ground. Either stay here or open your arms upward if that feels nice. Press your left fingertips to the ground, take a big inhale and open your body toward your right, lifting your right arm up. Gaze upward if you'd like. Bring your fingertips to the ground on either side of your front foot. Shift your hips back toward your back heel and relax

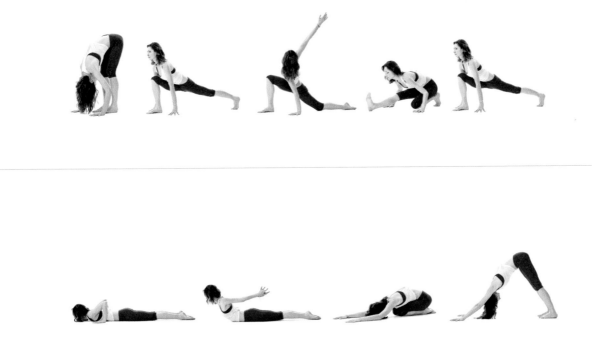

your torso over your front leg for your runner's stretch. Sway your torso side to side. Crawl yourself back to low lunge. Press your fingertips on the ground and lift your hips up for your single leg forward bend. Relax your torso over your front leg. Sway a bit side to side. When you're ready, sink your hips back to low lunge. Take a big inhale and lift up to high lunge. Exhale back to low lunge.

Press your palms on the ground on either side of your front foot and step back to plank. Soften your elbows and lower down to your belly. Interlace your hands behind you and open up your chest. Sway a bit here if that feels nice. When you're ready, soften back to your belly. Press your palms on the ground and sink your hips back to child's pose. Rest here for a few long, deep breaths. When you're ready, lift your hips, press your palms on the ground, take a big inhale, and lift up and back to down dog.

Repeat this movement phrase on the other side.

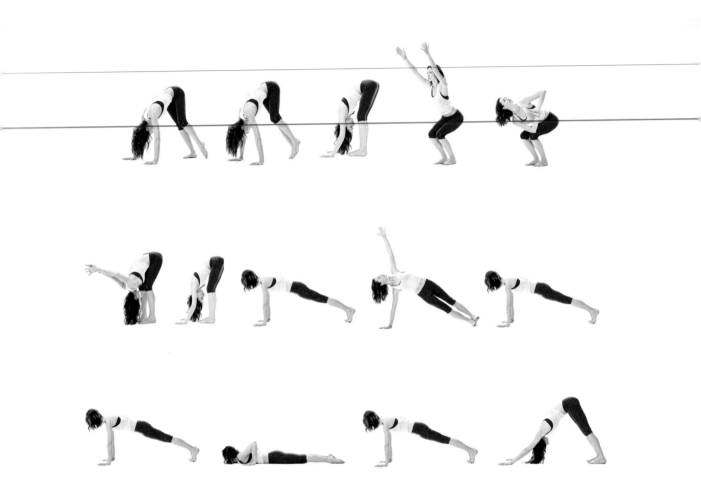

Walk your feet up to your hands and come into a standing forward bend. Sink your hips, take a big inhale, and lift yourself up into chair. Press your palms together, exhale, and twist to your left side, pressing your right elbow outside your left knee. Take a big inhale and come back to center. Exhale and twist to your right side. Inhale back to chair. Exhale and relax your torso over your legs, interlacing your hands behind you. Hang here for a few long, deep breaths. Release your hands, soften your knees, and press your palms to the ground. Step back to plank. Lift your hips and shift your weight onto your right hand and the outside edge of your right foot, take a big inhale, and open up into a side plank. If you want more stability, soften your right shin to the ground for support. Hang here for a few breaths. When you're ready, come back to center and go for the other side. When you're ready, come back to center. Soften your elbows and lower down to your belly. Press through your palms back up to plank and lift your hips up and back to down dog.

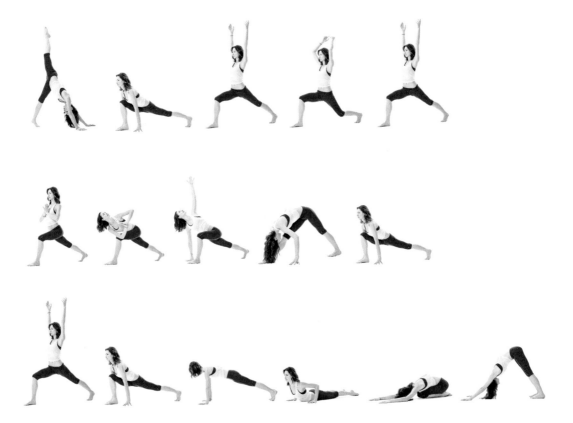

Take a big inhale and lift your right leg up to down dog split. Open your hips and shoulders if that feels nice. Exhale and step your foot between your hands to low lunge. Press down through your legs, take a big inhale, and lift up into high lunge. Exhale and soften a bit here. Inhale back to your high lunge. Exhale and soften a bit here. One more time, inhale up to high lunge. Exhale and press your palms together and bring your thumbs to your heartbeat. Take a big inhale and lift. Exhale and twist to your left side, bringing your right elbow outside your left leg. Open your arms, bringing your right fingertips to the ground inside your front foot and opening your left arm up. Gaze upward if you want to. Bring your fingertips of both hands to the ground on either side of your front foot. Take a big inhale, lift your hips up, and relax your torso over your front leg. Sway a bit here if that feels nice. Soften your knees back to low lunge. Take a big inhale and lift up to high lunge. Exhale back to low lunge, press your palms on the ground, and step back to plank. Soften your knees to the ground and sink your hips to up dog. If this doesn't feel nice on your lower back, soften your elbows to open your middle and upper back. Shift your hips back to your heels to child's pose. Rest here for a few long, deep breaths. When you're ready, lift your hips, press your palms on the ground, take a big inhale, and lift up and back to down dog.

Repeat this movement phrase on the other side.

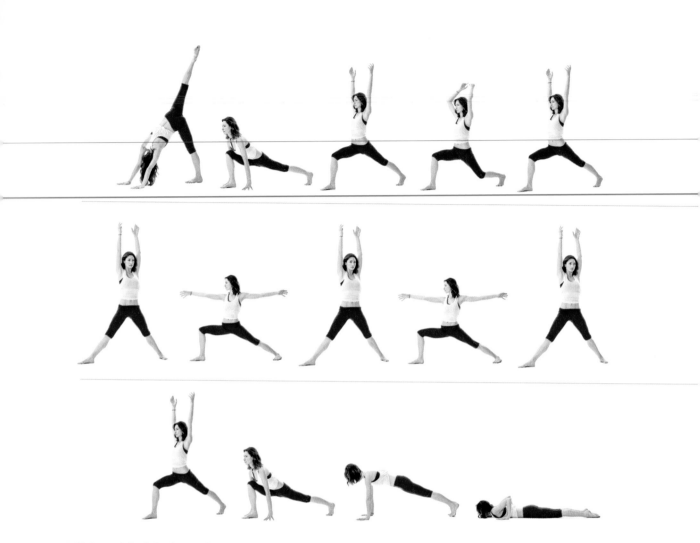

Take a big inhale and lift your right leg up to down dog split. Open your hips and shoulders if that feels nice. Exhale and step your foot between your hands to low lunge. Press down through your legs, take a big inhale, and lift up into high lunge. Exhale and soften a bit here. Inhale back to high lunge. Exhale and soften a bit here. One more time, inhale up to high lunge. Exhale and twist to your left and open your arms out to your sides. Inhale back to high lunge. Twice more like that, exhale and twist left, opening your arms wide, inhale back to high lunge. One more time, big exhale and twist left, inhale and lift back to high lunge. Open to warrior 2. Ground your back heel down, bend your front knee over your front foot, and open your arms out to your sides. Hang here for a few long, deep breaths.

Take a big inhale and lift your hips and arms up overhead. Exhale and soften back to warrior 2. Twice more like that, big inhale and lift. Easy exhale and soften. One more time, big inhale and lift. Easy exhale and soften. Tip back and reverse

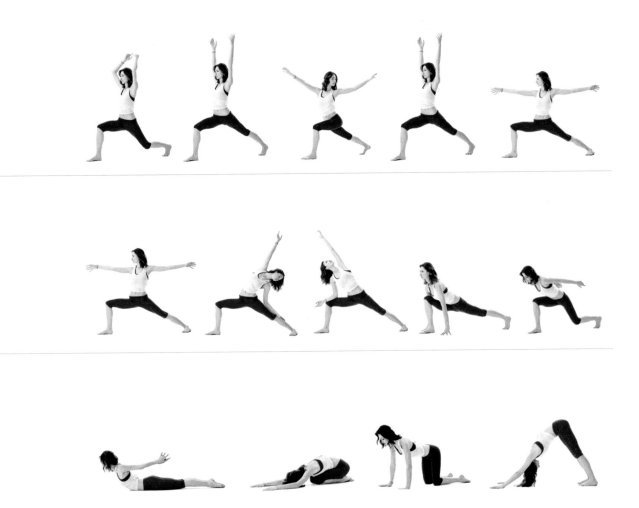

your warrior, sliding your left hand gently down your back leg and open your right arm up. Tip forward to your extended side angle, pressing your right forearm on your thigh and your left arm up and overhead. Roll your torso open if that feels nice. When you're ready, press your fingertips to the ground on either side of your front foot and come into low lunge. Push down through your legs, take a big inhale, and lift up to your high lunge. Exhale back down to low lunge, plant your palms on the ground, and step back to plank. Soften your elbows and lower down to your belly. Interlace your hands behind your back, take a big inhale, and lift your chest up. When you're ready, relax back down to your belly. Press your palms on the ground and shift your hips back to rest on your heels for child's pose. Hang here for a few long, deep breaths. Come onto all fours, tuck your toes, take a big inhale, and lift your hips up and back to down dog.

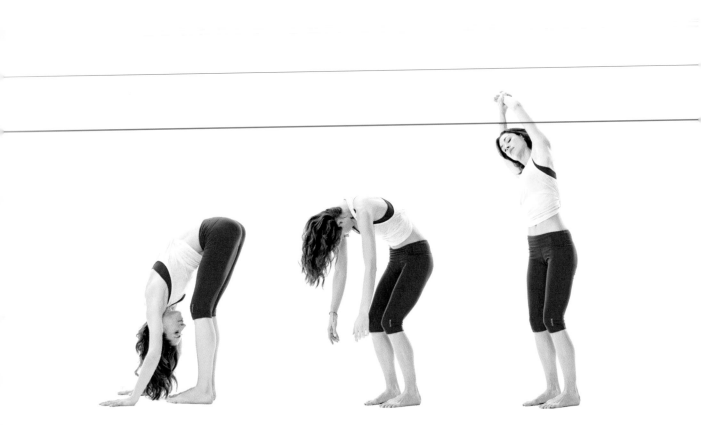

Walk your hands to your heels so you arrive in a standing forward bend at the back of your mat. Soften your knees and hang here for a few long, deep breaths. When you're ready, round up to stand one notch at a time. Once you make it up, take a big inhale and float your arms out and up. Grab ahold of your left wrist with your right hand. Soften here. Take a big inhale and lift up and over toward your right

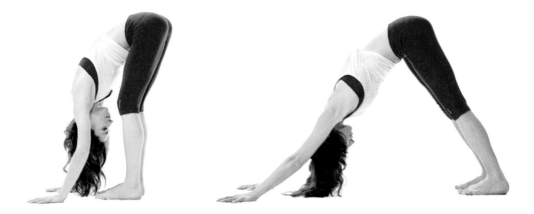

side. Roll around a bit here if that feels good. Come back to your center and go for the other side. When you're ready, come back to center, take a big inhale, and lift up. Exhale and soften your torso over your legs. Soften your knees and walk your hands back out to down dog.

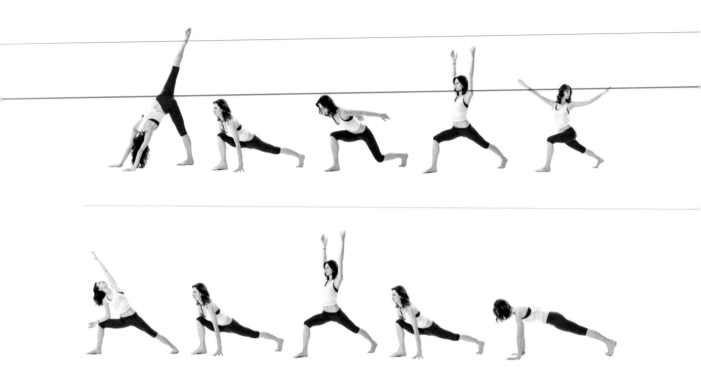

Take a big inhale and lift your right leg up and back to down dog split. Open up your hips if that feels nice for you. Exhale and step your foot through to low lunge. Press down through your legs and inhale up to high lunge. Exhale and twist to your left side and let your arms open wide. Inhale back to high lunge and open to warrior 2, spinning your back heel down so your toes point toward your front leg, and sink your hips. Bend your front knee over your front foot and open your arms out to your sides. Relax your head, neck, and shoulders. Breathe here for a few moments. Let the inhales lift you up a bit and the exhales soften you a bit more. Take a big inhale and lift your hips and arms up. Exhale and soften back to warrior 2. Take a big inhale and tip your torso back to reverse warrior, sliding your back hand gently down your back leg, and lift your opposite arm up. Tip forward into extended side angle, pressing your top forearm on your thigh and your opposite arm overhead. Roll your torso

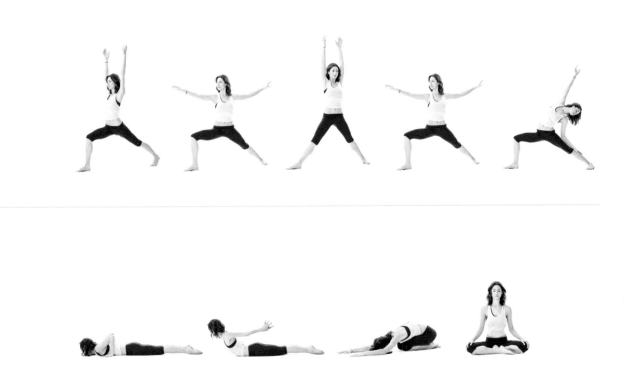

open if that feels good. Press your fingertips to the ground on either side of your front foot, and sink your hips to low lunge. Take a big inhale and lift up to high lunge. Exhale back to low lunge, press your palms on the ground, and press back to plank. Soften your elbows and lower down to your belly. Interlace your hands behind you, take a big inhale, and lift your chest up a bit. When you're ready, relax back to your belly. Press your palms on the ground next to your chest and shift your hips to your heels for child's pose. Rest here for a few moments.

Come up to sit comfortably. Close your eyes and rest your attention on your breath. Stay here with your breath for a few moments. Notice any sensations as they come and go. If you notice your attention drifting or shifting anywhere, guide your attention back to your breath.

Repeat the phrase on the other side. Stay easy with your breath.

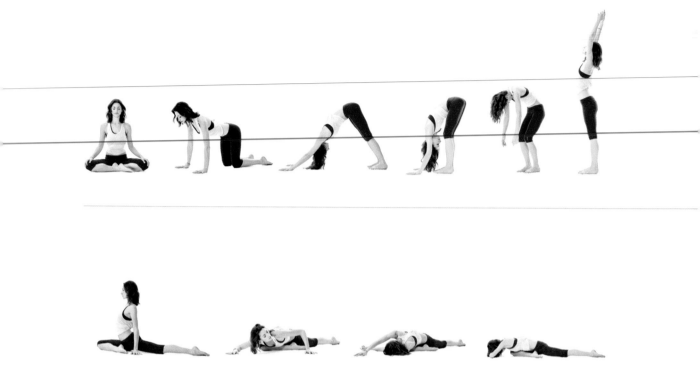

From seated, when you're ready, come onto all fours, tuck your toes, take a big inhale, and lift your hips up and back to down dog. Sway a bit here. When you're ready, walk your feet up to your hands gently and come into a standing forward bend, relaxing your torso over your legs. Round up to stand one notch at a time. When you make it up, take a big inhale and float your arms out and up. Press your palms together, close your eyes, and bring your thumbs to your heartbeat. Soften here for a few long, deep breaths. When you're ready, open your eyes. Shift your weight onto your right leg and hug your left shin into your chest. Roll around here. Press the bottom of your left foot into your right upper thigh, or, if it's more comfortable, press your toes on the ground so the bottom of your foot is connected to your right calf. Either press your thumbs into your heartbeat and lift your chest or open your arms up overhead for your tree. Hang here for a few long, deep breaths. Let your body sway a bit if that feels nice. When you're ready, hug your shin back into your chest and place your foot back down so both feet are on the ground and go for the other side, coming back to stand when you're finished.

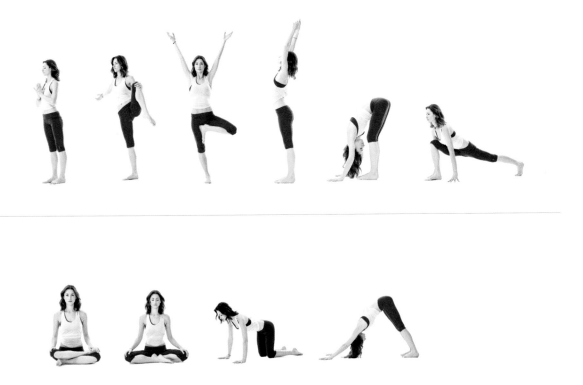

Take a big inhale and float your arms out and up. Exhale and soften back into your standing forward bend. Soften your knees and step your right leg back to low lunge. Soften your hips here. Slide your right foot over toward your left hand and relax your shin on the ground. Move your shin around a bit to find a comfortable place where you feel a nice opening in your hips and can breathe easily and freely. Either hang here upright, or relax your torso forward over your front shin. Feel free to explore, walking your hands around to one side and then the other to find a nice place to relax. Hang here for several long, deep breaths. Bring your torso back upright; staying seated, lean into your front hip, and swing your back leg in front of you. Stack your ankles on top of your knees, and if that doesn't feel nice for you, slide your left leg in front of your right leg and sit easy here. Bring your hands behind you for support. Take a big inhale and lean back. Either stay here or walk yourself forward, exploring around to one side and then the other if that feels nice. When you're ready, bring yourself back upright. Close your eyes and draw your attention inward. Hang here for several, long, deep breaths. Gently crawl yourself out onto all fours, tuck your toes, take a big inhale, and lift up and back to down dog.

Repeat the phrase on the other side. Stay easy with your breath.

NO PAIN = LOTS OF GAIN

Contrary to what we have been ingrained with in our lives, when we work and find ways of being that are pain-free, we experience a lot of gain. If you ever experience tweaking, pain, or a sensation that isn't simply your body working well for you, back away from the movement and come into a place that is comfortable. Don't worry if your movement looks the same or different from a picture or someone else's. The most important thing to keep in mind is to stay easy in a pain-free zone. You won't get ahead by harming your joints or pushing to the point of breaking. The goal is to sensitize yourself to how you feel, so you can get really good at feeling your way through the movements—and through the rest of your life. The more you prioritize feeling, the more you'll be able to accomplish with less effort.

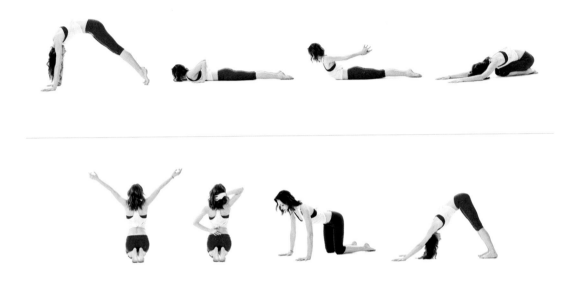

From down dog, round out to plank. Soften your elbows and lower down to your belly. Interlace your hands behind you, take a big inhale, and lift your torso up. When you're ready, relax back to your belly. Press your palms on the ground and shift your hips back to your heels. Rest in child's pose for a few long, deep breaths. Come up to sit on your heels. Take a big inhale and float your arms out and up. Relax your left arm down and around your back as you soften your right elbow. Link your hands together if that's easy. If that doesn't feel good, keep your hands apart on your back. Lean back if that feels good. Hang here for a few long, deep breaths and move around a bit, however it feels nice for you to open up here. When you're ready, relax your arms and repeat on the other side. Come back onto all fours, tuck your toes, and take a big inhale to lift your hips up and back to down dog.

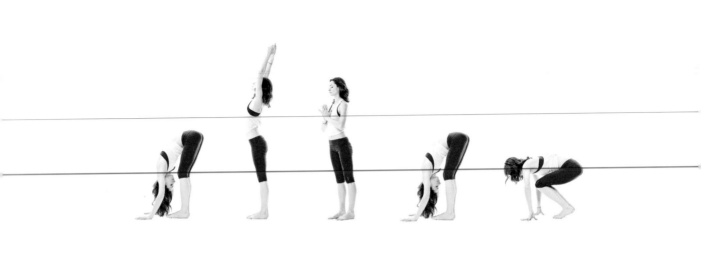

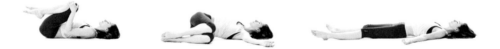

From down dog, take an easy stroll up to the top of your mat to standing forward bend. Relax your head and neck here and sway a bit. Roll up to stand one notch at a time. When you make it up, float your arms out and up. Press your palms together, close your eyes, and bring your thumbs to your heartbeat. Soften here for a moment. Soften your knees. Relax your head, neck, and shoulders. Sway a bit side to side. Take a big inhale and lift your arms up, opening your eyes if you like. Exhale and soften over your legs. Press your palms on the ground, shift some weight into your arms, and come to an easy squat. Open up here, lifting your arm and rolling your torso side to side if that feels nice. When you're ready, bring your hands behind you for support and come to sit.

Bring the bottoms of your feet together and let your knees open out to your sides. Press your hands behind you on the ground for support. Take a big inhale, lean back, and open up here. Either stay here if this feels nice or crawl your torso forward to relax. Hang here for several deep breaths. Roll yourself down to lie on your back. To be easy on your back, bring your knees along with you for the ride. If you'd like to take a gentle twist, let your knees drift to one side and rest for a few

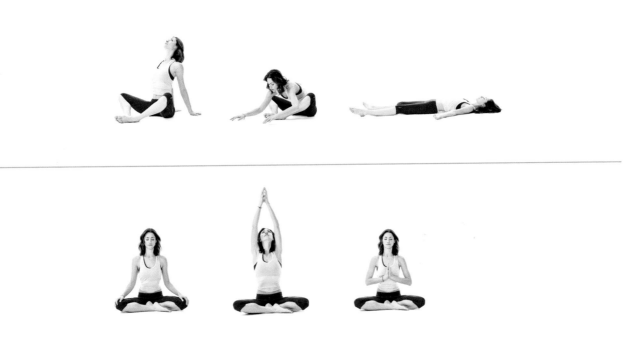

deep breaths. Open your arms out to the side to relax. Try the same on the other side. When you are ready to relax, stretch out a bit, close your eyes, and rest for several breaths.

When you're ready to come out of this, invite some more air back in. Open your eyes if you'd like. Roll your wrists and ankles around if that feels nice. Make your way up to sit easily and comfortably. Take your time. Come to a simple, easy seat. Close your eyes and draw your attention back inward. Take a big inhale and float your arms out and up. Press your palms together and bring your thumbs to your heartbeat. Soften here for a moment. Take a big inhale through your nose. Long exhale through your mouth. Twice more like that, big inhale, long exhale. One more time, big inhale, long exhale. When you are ready, relax your hands on your thighs and gently open your eyes.

You did it! Great job. I hope you feel energized and focused and excited to continue practicing. Enjoy!

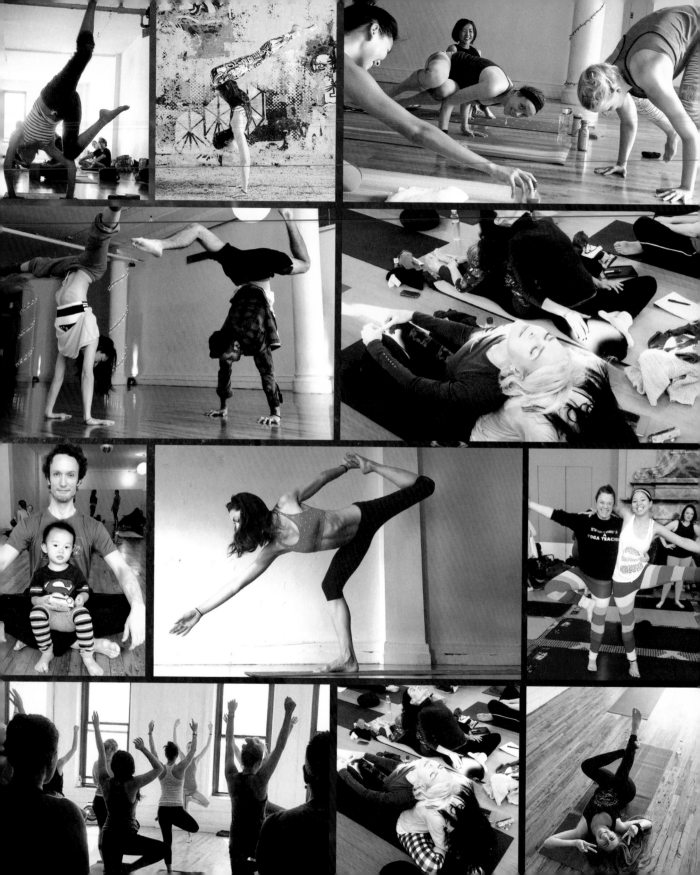

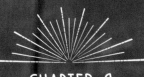

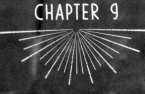

CHAPTER 9

CORE

This routine is designed to bring awareness and strengthen your core. You'll be moving in all directions to work every area of your middle, building strength and the ability to move more easily and naturally. Stay with your breath, and allow your body and mind to relax as you move. Use only the energy you need to get through the movements. Move through this a few times a week to gain a nice range of motion and ease of body and mind.

It's useful to keep in mind that you'll be building a strong core with all the movements here. When you move naturally, softening as you move, in the easiest way possible, through simple and challenging movements, you are building a tremendous amount of strength. This workout is far superior to isolated abdominal exercises. This core-focused routine gets you moving everything, all together, putting together strong movement phrases to give you a nice impact.

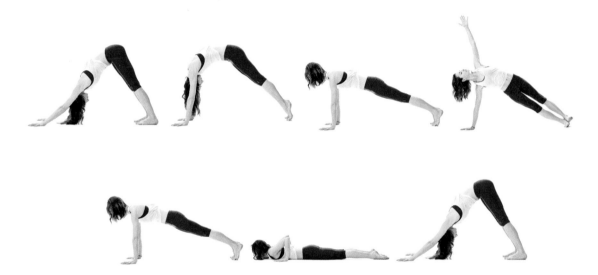

Come into down dog. Move a bit here to get comfortable. Round out to plank. Lift your hips, shift your weight onto your right hand and the outside edge of your right foot, and open your body to your left. If you want some more stability, soften your right shin to the ground for support. Hang here for a few long, deep breaths. Come back to center and go for the other side. When you're ready, come back to center. Soften your elbows and lower down to your belly. In one piece, press right back up and back to down dog.

Repeat the movement phrase two more times, moving easily with your breath.

RESIST THE URGE TO FLEX

It's a common misunderstanding that flexing and engaging build strength. Observing some of the strongest creatures on the planet, we learn a great deal about strength and power as it relates to the core. Flip on the Nature Channel and observe a lion climbing a tree. The lion doesn't prepare to climb the tree by doing a bunch of crunches or flexing her muscles. She uses the least amount of effort possible. The lion's power comes from exploration. She gets to know what she is capable of and her body really well. Through that knowing, she is able to expand what she is capable of and build strength. The magic is the appearance of effortless strength and grace.

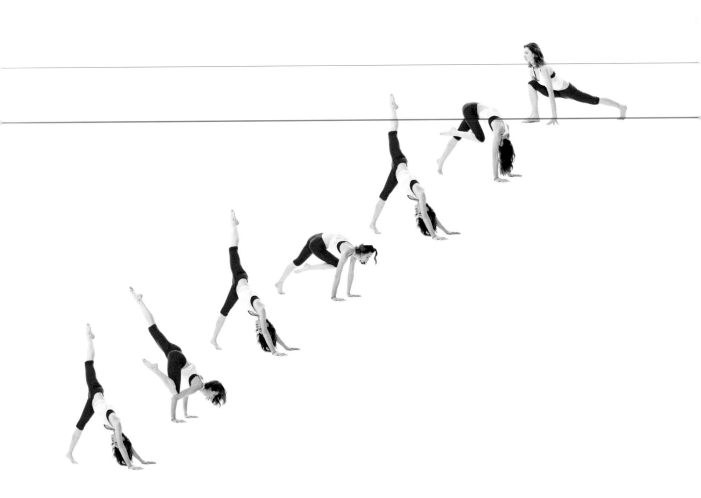

Take a big inhale and lift your right leg up and back to down dog split. Arc your knee high and around to your right upper arm. Look forward and lean forward. Take a big inhale and lift your leg back to down dog split. Arc your knee across your body to your left upper arm. Make a shelf out of your arm here. Look forward and lean forward. When you're ready, lift your leg back to down dog split. Step your foot between your hands to low lunge. Take a big inhale and lift up to high lunge. Exhale back down to low lunge. Plant your palms on the ground and step back to plank. Lift up your hips,

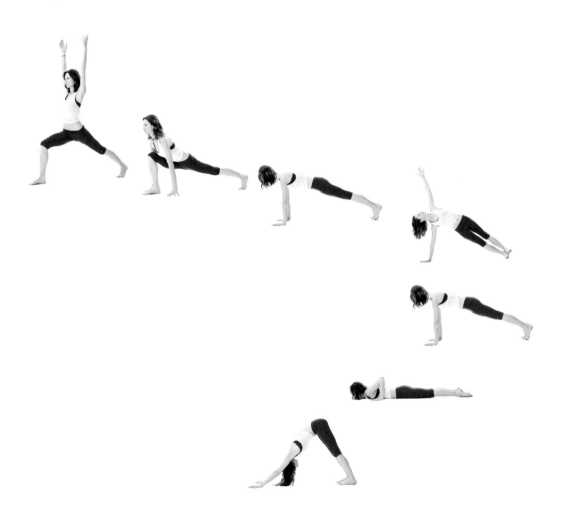

shift your weight onto your right hand and the outside edge of your right foot, and open your body to your left side. If you want some more stability, soften your right shin to the ground for support. Hang here for a few long, deep breaths. Come back to center and go for the other side. When you're ready, come back to center. Soften your elbows and lower to your belly. In one piece, press right back up and back to down dog.

Repeat this movement phrase twice on each side.

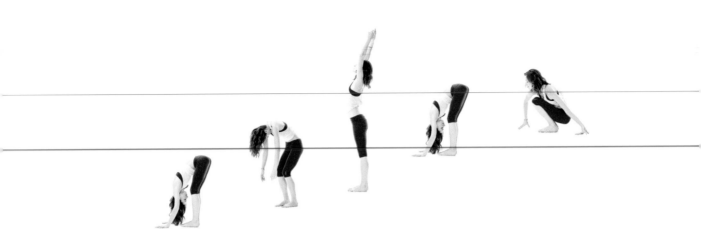

Walk your feet up to your hands and come into standing forward bend. Soften your knees a bit here and relax your torso over your legs. Roll up to stand one notch at a time. When you make it up, take a big inhale and float your arms out and up overhead. Exhale and relax back to standing forward bend. Press your palms to the ground and soften your knees, coming into a squat. Bring your hands behind you and come to sit easily.

Lift your legs in front of you with your knees soft for your boat. If this is too much on your lower back, place your hands or forearms on the ground behind you for support. Lower your body halfway down toward the ground and lift back up, keeping your head, neck, and shoulders relaxed. Repeat this 10 times, moving with your breath. Lower halfway down and on your right side with your arms across to your left for a boat twist. Lift back up. Twist in the opposite direction and roll through this about 10 times with your breath. Lower down and open your arms behind you, pressing your lower back toward the ground. Take a big inhale here to open up. Exhale and hug your knees while relaxing on your back.

Rock a bit side to side if that feels good. Rock gently forward and back to come up to sit. Press your hands on the ground in front of you for support and lift up into a standing forward bend, keeping your knees soft. Relax your head and neck here. Round up to stand one notch at a time. Take a big inhale and float your arms out and up overhead. Exhale and soften back into standing forward bend. Press your palms on the ground and step back to plank. Lift up to side plank on your right hand. If you want some more stability, soften your right shin to the ground for support. Hang here for a few long, deep breaths. Go for the other side. Soften your elbows and lower down to your belly. In one piece, press right back up to plank and then back to down dog.

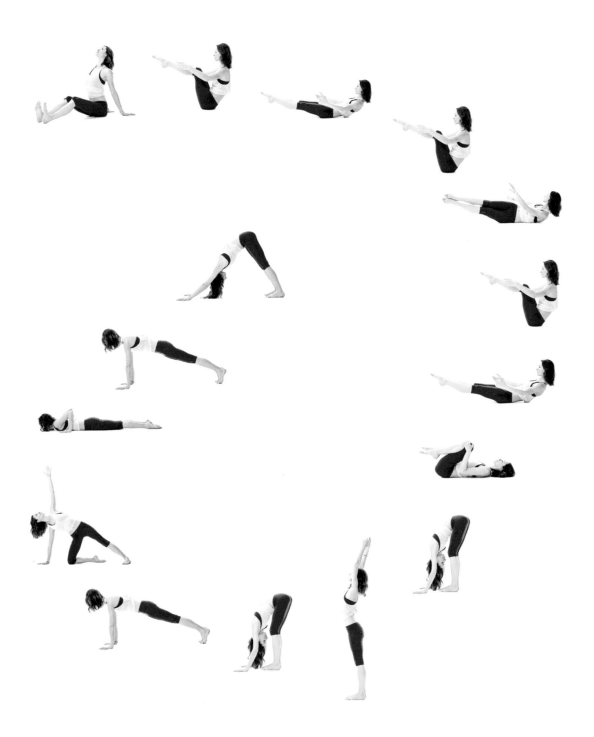

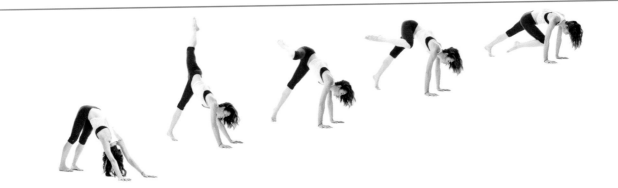

Take a big inhale and float your right leg up and back to down dog split. Open your hips and belly here if that feels nice. Arc your knee high and around to your right upper arm. Look forward and lean forward. Inhale right back up to down dog split. Arc your knee down and across to your left upper arm. Look forward and lean forward. Inhale your leg back to down dog split.

Let's go for some hip rolls. From down dog split, arc your knee high and around to your right upper arm; keep it moving across to the left, sweep it back open to the right and up and back to down dog split. Now bring your knee down and across to your left upper arm, open right, up and back to down dog split. One more time all of that, high and around right, across left, open right, up and back to down dog split. Last round, down and across left, open right, up and back to down dog split.

Exhale and step your right foot forward to low lunge. Inhale up to high lunge. Exhale back to low lunge. Plant your palms on the ground and step back to plank. Soften your elbows and lower down to your belly. Press back to plank and lift up and back to down dog.

Repeat this and the previous movement phrases (starting with walking up to standing forward bend) on the other side.

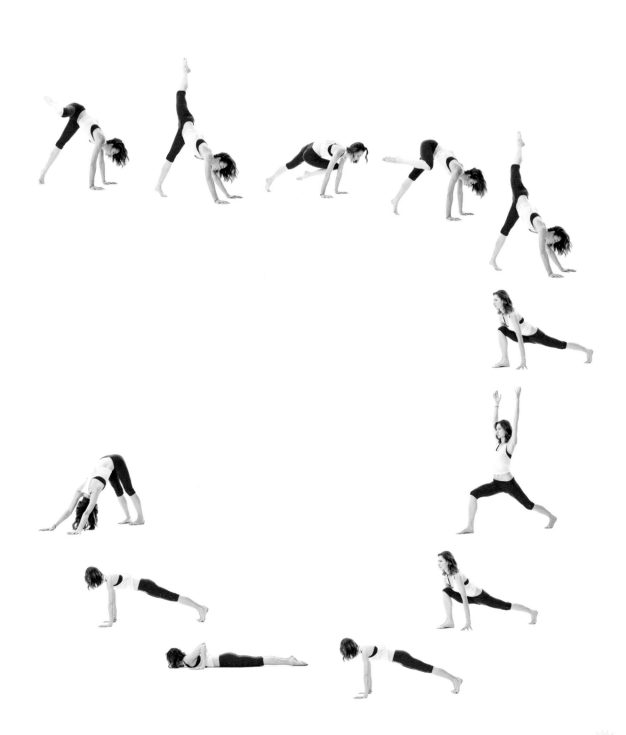

KEEP IT
ROLLIN'

For the hip rolls, it's important not to rush through the movements or treat them like a calisthenic exercise. The purpose of the hip rolls is to move your entire body all together and easily in many directions. These movements build strength in your core and entire body, while helping you maintain a healthy range of mobility. Enjoy the rolls!

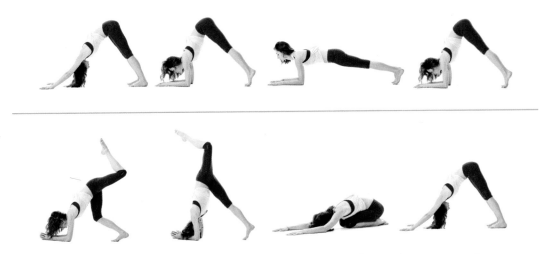

From down dog, soften your elbows and come into a down dog on your forearms. Hang here for a few long, deep breaths. Walk your feet out into a forearm plank. Hang here for a few long deep breaths. Walk your feet back up to down dog on your forearms. Take a big inhale and lift your left leg up, lifting your hips and belly. Exhale and soften back down. Repeat on your right side. When you're ready, soften your knees to the ground and relax in child's pose. Rest here for a few long, deep breaths. When you're ready, lift your hips, tuck your toes, take a big inhale, and lift up and back to down dog.

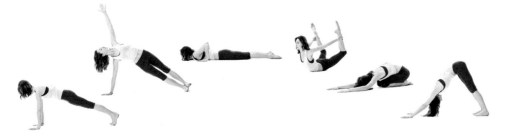

From down dog, roll out to plank. Hang here for 20 long, deep breaths. When the going gets tough, stay easy, sway a bit side to side, and relax. Lift up to side plank for 10 breaths. If you want some more stability, soften your right shin to the ground for support. Then go for the other side. Come back to center. Soften your elbows and lower down to your belly and relax. Bend your knees, grab ahold of your ankles, and lift up into bow. Rock a bit here if that feels nice. If this hurts your lower back, don't do it; just stay and relax on your belly. When you're ready, relax back to your belly and rest here for a few moments. Press your palms on the ground and shift your hips back to child's pose. Rest here for a moment. When you're ready, lift your hips up a bit, press your palms on the ground, and lift up and back to down dog.

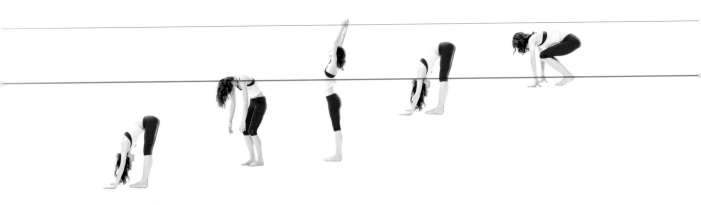

Take an easy stroll up to the top of your mat, coming into standing forward bend. Roll up to stand one notch at a time. When you make it up, take a big inhale and float your arms out and up. Exhale and relax over your legs. Press your palms into the ground and bring yourself into a squat. Bring your hands on the ground behind you and bring yourself to sit. Bring the bottoms of your feet together and lean back a bit to open up. Either stay here if that feels nice or relax your torso forward for a few breaths. When you're ready, roll down to lie on your back, bringing your knees along with you for the ride. Press the bottoms of your feet on the ground next to your hips. Relax your arms down by your sides and lift up into bridge. Hang here for a few long, deep breaths. Relax back down. Press your palms on the ground next to your ears, and lift up into wheel. If this doesn't feel good, relax down. Hang here for several long, deep breaths. Relax back down and rest for a few deep breaths. Hug your knees into your chest, then bring your legs to your right side and open your arms out to your sides, coming into a twist. Hang here for a few long, deep breaths. When you're ready, go for the other side. Stretch out and relax for several long, deep breaths.

Bring yourself up easily to sit. Relax your hands on your thighs and draw your attention inward. Take a big inhale and float your arms out and up. Press your palms together, close your eyes, and bring your thumbs to your heartbeat. Soften here for a moment. Take a big inhale through your nose. Long exhale out through your mouth. Twice more just like that. Big inhale, long exhale. Once more, big inhale, long exhale. Relax your hands gently back on your thighs and when you're ready, open your eyes.

I hope you feel strong, energetic, and ready to climb any tree you desire!

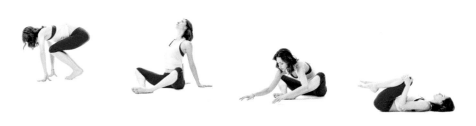

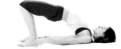

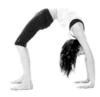

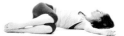

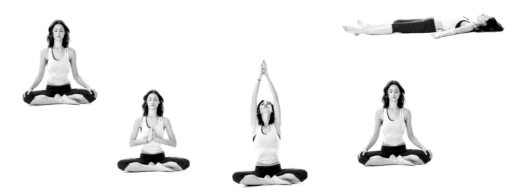

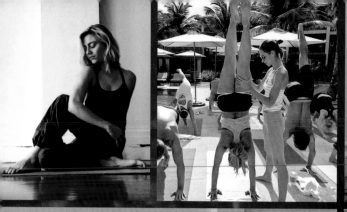
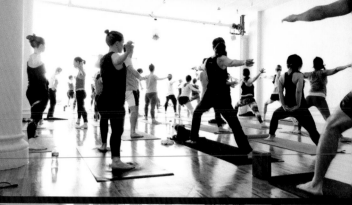
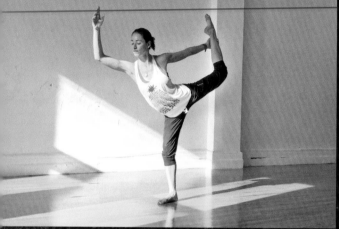
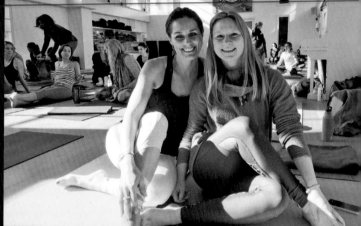
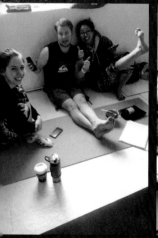
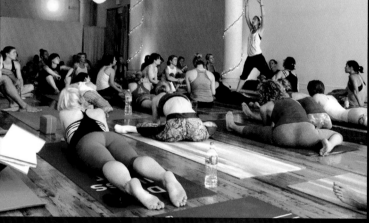
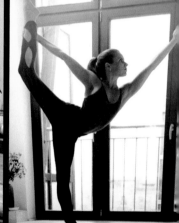
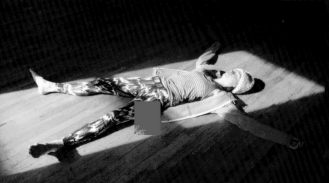
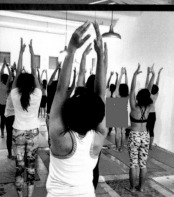
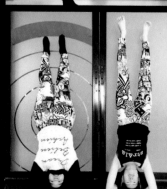

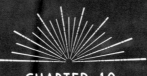

CHAPTER 10

GENTLE

This routine is designed to be very gentle and restorative. The movements will softly open the body, release tension, and calm the mind into deep relaxation. Take your time in each movement, and stay easy with your breath as you flow gently to gain a nice, relaxing feeling.

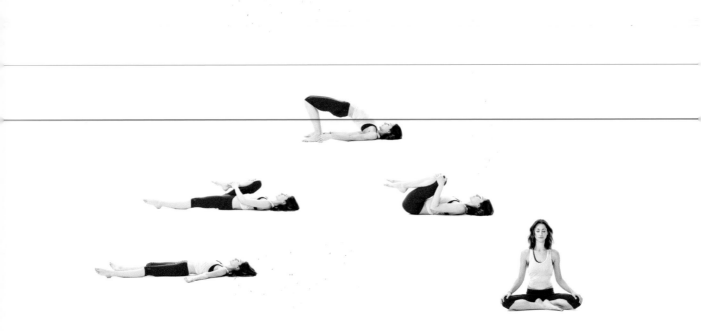

Start lying down comfortably. Bring your attention to your breath. Let your inhales and exhales deepen and come from your belly. Hug your right shin into your chest. Roll your shin around to get into your hips a bit. Hang here for a few long, deep breaths. When you're ready, bring your leg back to center, relax it down to meet your left leg, and go for the other side. Hug both knees into your chest and place your feet on the ground next to your hips.

Press your arms on the ground alongside your torso and lift your hips up into a bridge. Hang here for a few long, deep breaths. Ease yourself gently back to the ground and relax for a few deep breaths. Hug your knees into your chest and rock a bit side to side if that feels good. Take your time and find an easy way to come up to sit. Relax your hands on your thighs, close your eyes, and draw your attention inward.

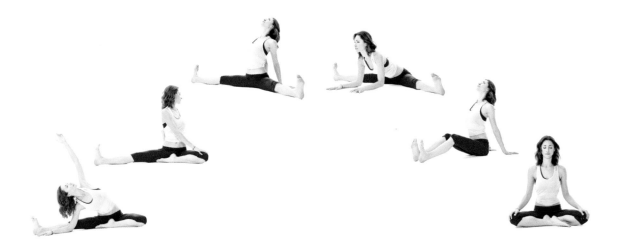

From seated, extend your right leg out toward the side. Press your right hand on the ground inside your right leg. Soften your elbow and lean over to your right side, opening your left arm up overhead. Hang here for a few long, deep breaths. When you're ready, bring yourself back up and take an easy twist, pressing your right hand on your left thigh and your left fingertips on the ground behind you for support. Take a big inhale and lift up. Exhale and twist around a little farther. Stay with this for a few breaths and bring yourself back to center. Try the movements on your left side.

Open your legs out to your sides. Press your fingertips behind you for support. Take a big inhale and lift up your torso. Either stay here if this feels nice or walk yourself forward. Let your torso sway side to side if that feels nice. Stay here for several long, deep breaths. When you're ready, bring yourself back up. Bring your legs out in front of you and together. Put a soft bend in your knees to take the pressure off your hamstrings. Press your fingertips on the ground behind you for support. Take a big inhale and open up your body here. Either stay here or relax your torso forward. Sway a bit side to side. When you're ready, bring yourself back to sitting upright.

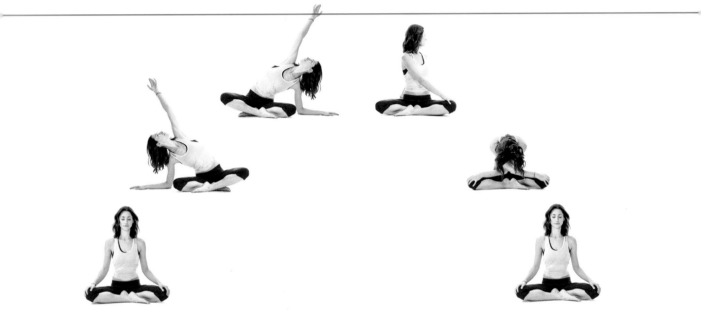

From sitting, close your eyes and relax your hands on your thighs. Bring your attention back to your breath. Lean toward your right side, pressing your right forearm on the ground beside you for support. Soften your elbow and arch your left arm up and overhead. Hang here for a few long, deep breaths. When you're ready, come back to center and lean over toward your other side. Take a big inhale and lift your right arm up. Bring yourself back to center. Twist toward your left, pressing your right hand on top of your left thigh. Bring your left fingertips behind you for support. Take a big inhale and lift up. Exhale and twist around a little more. Bring your left arm up and around and grab hold of your right knee with your left hand. Relax your torso forward and roll around a bit here if that feels nice. When you're ready, bring yourself back upright and go for the other side. Come back to an easy neutral seat. Close your eyes, relax your hands on your thighs, and draw your attention back inward. Hang here for a few breaths.

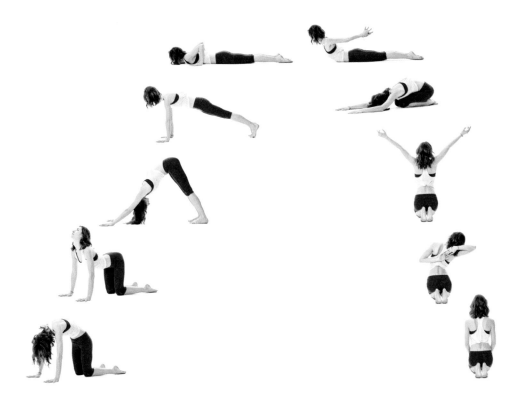

When you're ready, gently crawl out onto all fours. Move your torso with your breath, however it feels good for you. When you're ready, tuck your toes, take a big inhale, and lift your hips up and back to down dog. Move around here a bit to open up. Round out to plank. Soften your elbows and gently lower down to your belly. Interlace your hands behind you, take a big inhale, and lift up a bit. Relax your torso back down. Press your palms on the ground and shift your hips back to your heels to rest in child's pose. Hang here for a few deep breaths. Come up to sit on your heels.

Take a big inhale and float your arms out and up overhead. Soften your elbows; drop your left arm down and around your back. Bend your right elbow so your hand comes down your back, as well. If your hands hook together easily, hook them up. If not, no worries, keep some space between them so you're comfortable. Hang here for a few long, deep breaths. Move your torso around here however it feels good to you. Relax your arms and go for the other side. When you're ready, come back to your center, relax your hands on your thighs, and rest for a few deep breaths.

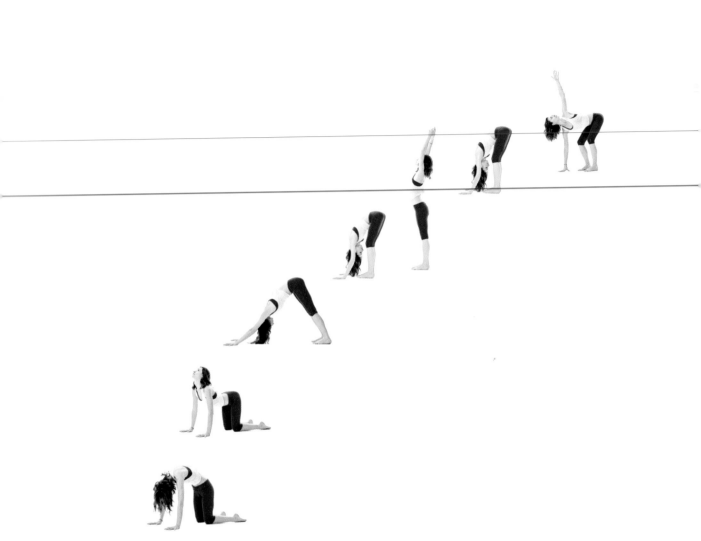

Gently come onto all fours. Roll your torso around here how it feels good for you. Tuck your toes and lift your hips up and back to down dog. Walk your feet up to your hands and come into a standing forward bend. Soften your knees and relax your head and neck here. Roll up to stand one notch at a time. Once you make it up, take a big inhale and float your arms up and overhead. As you exhale, relax your torso back over your legs. Press your right fingertips on the ground in front of your feet a bit. Soften your knees, take a big inhale, and open your left arm upward and open your body toward your left. Gaze upward if that feels nice for you. When you're ready, relax back to center and go for the other side.

   Soften your knees and step your left leg back to low lunge. Sink your hips here and move a bit side to side. When you're ready, soften your back knee down and

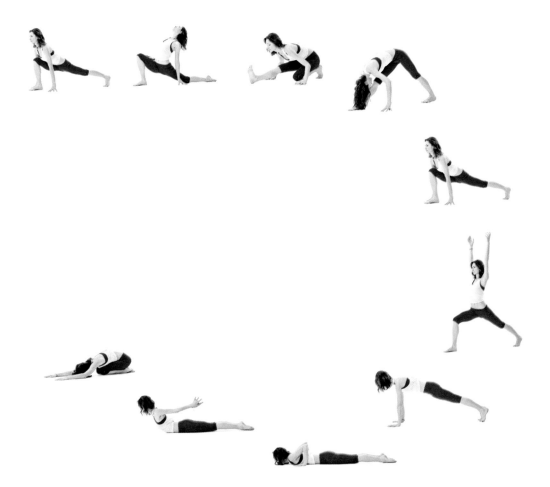

open your chest and arms up if you'd like. Hang here for a few deep breaths. Bring your fingertips to the ground and shift your hips back to sit on your back heel for your runner's stretch. Relax your torso over your front leg for a few deep breaths. Crawl yourself back to your low lunge, tuck your back toes, and lift your hips up to your single leg forward bend. Relax your torso over your front leg and hang here for a few deep breaths. Sink your hips back to low lunge. Press down through your legs and lift up to high lunge. Exhale back through low lunge, plant your palms back to the ground, and step back to plank. Soften your elbows and lower down to your belly. Interlace your hands behind you and open the front of your body for a few deep breaths. When you're ready, relax your body back down. Press your palms on the ground and sink your hips back to child's pose. Rest here for a few breaths.

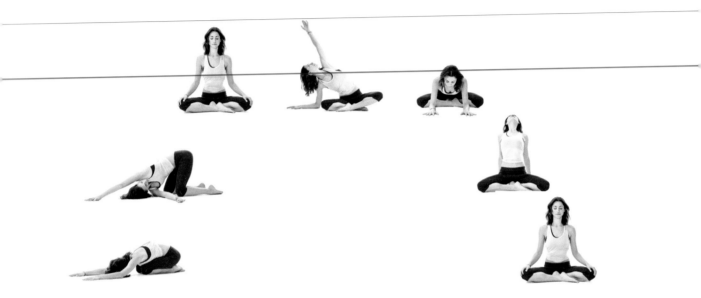

From child's pose, thread your right shoulder under your left, resting your right shoulder on the ground. Hang here for a few long, deep breaths. Come back to center and go for the other side. Come back to center and gently bring yourself to an easy seated position. Relax your hands on your thighs and draw your attention inward.

Staying easy in your body, lean to your right, resting your right hand and forearm on the ground beside you. Open your left arm up and over your head. Hang here for a few breaths, moving your body gently a bit to open things up. Come back up to the middle and go for the other side. Walk your hands forward and let your torso relax. Sway a bit here if that feels nice for you. When you are ready, gently bring yourself back up to the middle. Walk yourself forward a bit and relax your torso over your legs. Sway a bit here. Bring yourself back up to center. Press your fingertips behind you on the ground, take a big inhale, and lift your chest and hips up. As you exhale, relax to your center. Rest your hands on your thighs, close your eyes for a moment, guiding your attention back to your breath.

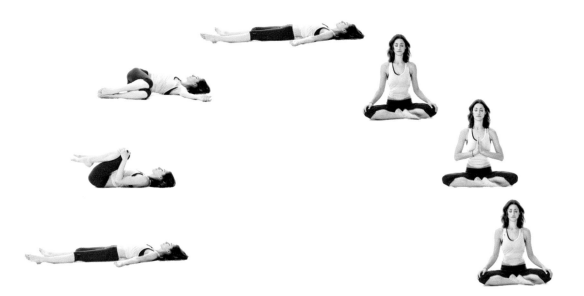

When you're ready, open your eyes and gently round down to lie on your back, bringing your knees along with you as you roll down. Hug your knees into your chest gently and rock a bit side to side if that feels good for you. Let your knees drift over to your left side and open your arms out to your sides. Hang here for a few long, deep breaths and go for the other side. Stretch out a bit and relax. Take a big inhale through your nose and long exhale out through your mouth. Rest here for a few moments. Gently bring yourself up to sit in the easiest way possible. Stay relaxed and soft as you move. Rest your palms on your thighs and draw your attention inward. Take a big inhale and float your arms out and up. Press your palms together and bring your thumbs to your heartbeat. Soften here for a moment. Take a big inhale through your nose. Long exhale out through your mouth. Twice more just like that. Big inhale, long exhale. Once more, big inhale, long exhale. Relax your hands gently back on your thighs and, when you're ready, open your eyes.

Great job! I hope you feel calm, relaxed, and rejuvenated.

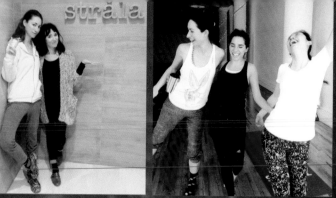
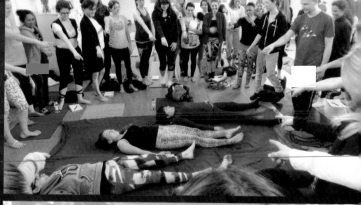
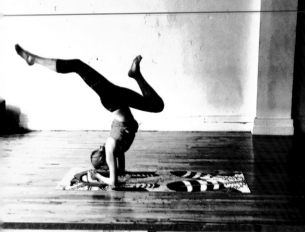
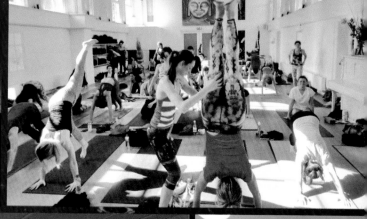
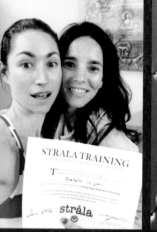
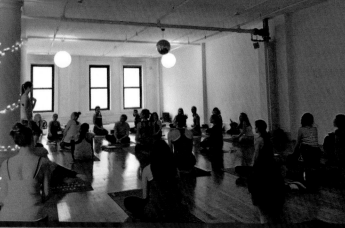
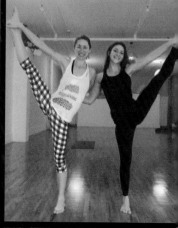
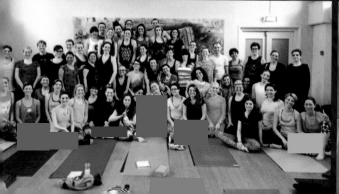
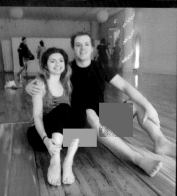
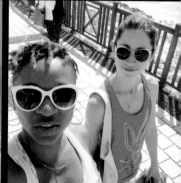

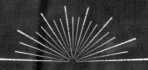

TARGET PRACTICES

There are a few simple routines to target everyday needs to improve how you feel. We all want to feel better, and these routines are designed to do just that, targeting specific moments where some support is beneficial. Feel free to practice these routines whenever and wherever.

WAKE UP

Too often our mornings are about jumping out of bed and racing into the day. We end up feeling constantly rushed and yet somehow always behind. Luckily we can do something to make for a better day. We just have to focus our energy so we don't get frazzled or overwhelmed by our to-do lists. This routine is designed to calm and focus your mind and to power up and open your body. I've been doing this for years, and it makes a huge difference. Just a few moments for yourself in the morning can shift everything. Bonus: you can do this in bed before you even get up. Rise and shine!

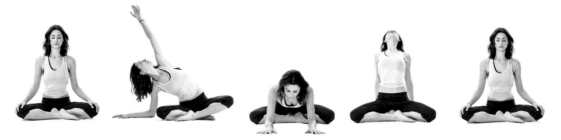

Start seated on your bed, however you can be comfortable. If you have a headboard or a wall that you can lean on, that's a nice option. If you feel comfortable sitting upright without support, that's great too. The most important thing is to be comfortable. Draw your attention inward. Watch your inhales and exhales as they come and go. If you notice your attention starting to drift, guide it back to your breath. Stay with this for a few moments.

Staying easy in your body, lean to your right, resting your right hand and forearm on the ground beside you. Open your left arm up and over your head. Hang here for a few breaths, moving your body gently a bit to open things up. Come back up to center and go for the other side. Walk your hands forward and let your torso relax. Sway a bit here if that feels nice for you. When you are ready, gently bring yourself back up to the middle. Press your fingertips behind you on the bed, take a big inhale, and lift your chest and hips up. As you exhale, relax to your middle. Rest your hands on your thighs and close your eyes for a moment, guiding your attention back to your breath.

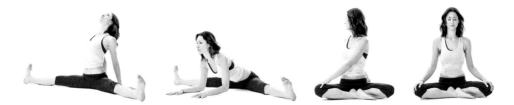

Open your legs, press your hands behind you on the bed, and take a big inhale to open up. Either stay here if this feels nice or walk yourself forward. Roll your torso around however it feels nice. When you're ready, bring yourself back upright and come into an easy seated position. Take a big inhale and lift your left arm up. Exhale and press your hand on your right thigh. Bring your right fingertips behind you for support. Take a big inhale and lift up a bit. Exhale and twist toward your right. Hang here for a few more deep breaths, repeating the movement, and go for the other side. When you're ready, bring yourself back to center.

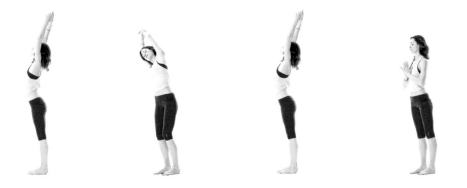

Bring yourself to the edge of your bed and place your feet on the floor. Press down on the bed with your hands and down through your legs to come up to stand. Take a big inhale and float your arms out and up. Grab ahold of your left wrist with your right hand. Take a big inhale and lift up and exhale to open over to your right side. Hang here for a few breaths. When you're ready, go for the other side. Bring yourself back to your center. Press your palms together, close your eyes, and bring your thumbs to your heartbeat. Soften here for a moment. Take a big inhale through your nose. Long exhale out through your mouth. Repeat twice more like that. Big inhale, long exhale. One more time, big inhale, long exhale. Relax your arms down by your sides, open your eyes, and open your eyes.

I hope you feel connected, refreshed, energized, and ready for an awesome day!

BETTER SLEEP

This routine is designed to calm any remaining tension in your body and mind so you can have a restful night's sleep. Just like the wake-up routine, you can practice this right from the comfort of your bed, so you are all set to be supercozy for the night. Stay easy with your breath and enjoy. Dream well!

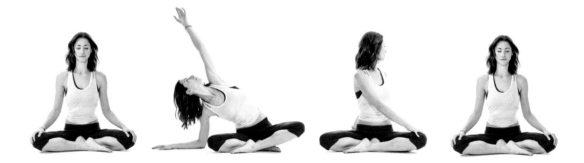

Get cozy in your bed. Sit up however you can be comfortable. Close your eyes and draw your attention inward. If you notice your attention wandering, guide it back to your breath. Hang here for a few long, deep breaths.

Staying easy in your body, lean to your right, resting your right hand and forearm on the bed beside you. Open your left arm and bring it up and over your head. Hang here for a few breaths, moving your body gently to open things up a bit. When you're ready, come back up to the middle and go for the other side, inhaling and lifting your right arm up. Bring your right arm down and press your right hand on top of your left thigh and your left hand on the bed behind you for support. Take a big inhale and lift your torso up. Twist toward your left, pressing your right hand on your left thigh. Exhale and twist a little farther around. Repeat this a few more times with your breath. When you're done, bring yourself back to the center. Go for the other side. When you're ready, come back to center. Rest your hands on your thighs and close your eyes for a moment, guiding your attention back to your breath.

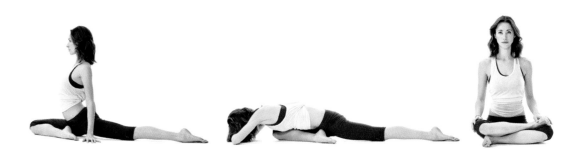

Sit into your right hip and bring your left leg behind you for pigeon. Get comfortable here. Try moving your right foot either closer toward or away from you to find a place where you feel a good opening in your hips and you can still breathe easily. Take a big inhale and open up a bit here. Exhale and walk yourself forward and relax on your bed. Hang here for several long, deep breaths. When you're ready, bring yourself back up, lean into your right hip, and bring your left leg around. Stack your ankles and knees on top of each other if that feels comfortable. If stacking isn't comfortable, bring your left leg to rest in front of your right leg. Hang here for a few breaths. If it feels good, relax your torso forward, walking your hands to one side and then the other. Bring yourself back upright and repeat the movements on your other side starting with pigeon.

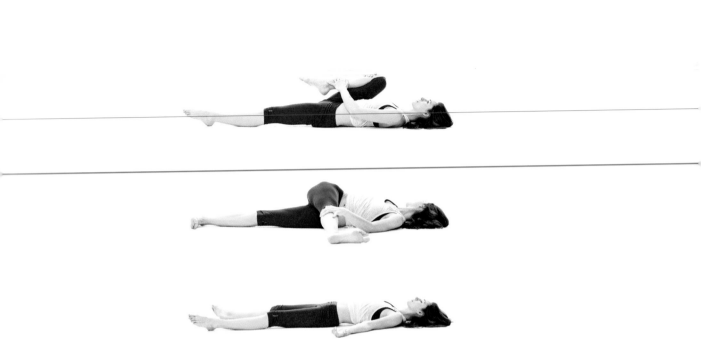

Lie down comfortably. Hug your right knee into your chest. Roll your leg around to gently open your hips a bit. Hang here for a few long, deep breaths. Rest your right leg across you toward your left side. Relax your left arm over your right leg and open your right arm out to your side. Hang in this twist for a few long, deep breaths. Come back to center and go for the other side. Come back to center—and you're lying down comfortably. Sweet dreams!

I hope you are drifting off to a wonderful night's sleep and feel fantastic and well rested in the morning.

WIND DOWN

This routine is designed to drop any stress and tension that latches on during the day. It's like a reset button for your day—separating part one (work, errands, meetings, and such) from part two (going out, hanging with friends, relaxing at home, or something else). So enjoy easing from one to the next and begin again with a fresh start . . . whatever your plans.

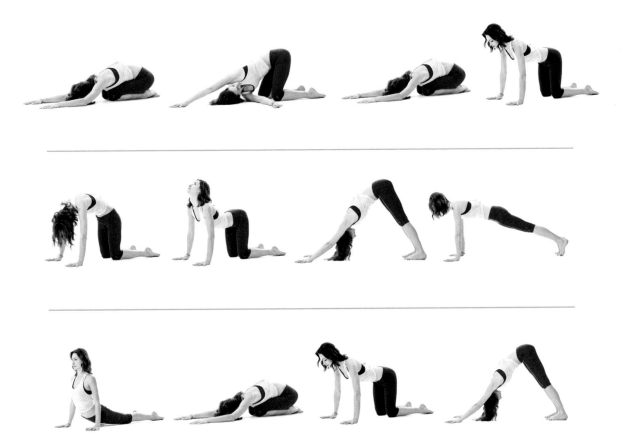

Come into child's pose. Relax your forehead on the ground and rest here for several long, deep breaths. Let your exhales be a little longer than your inhales. Lift your hips up a bit and thread your right arm under your left and relax your right shoulder on the ground. Hang here for several long, deep breaths. Let yourself move around however it feels good to get a nice opening in your shoulders. Come back through your center and go for the other side. Come back to child's pose and rest here for a few long, deep breaths.

Come onto all fours and roll your body around how it feels good to you, breathing deeply. Tuck your toes, take a big inhale, and lift up and back to down dog.

Tuck your chin and round out to plank. Soften your knees to the ground, sink your hips, and open your chest forward into up dog. Roll around here a bit if that feels good. Shift your hips to your heels for child's pose. Rest here for a few long, deep breaths. Come up to all fours, tuck your toes, and take a big inhale and lift up and back to down dog.

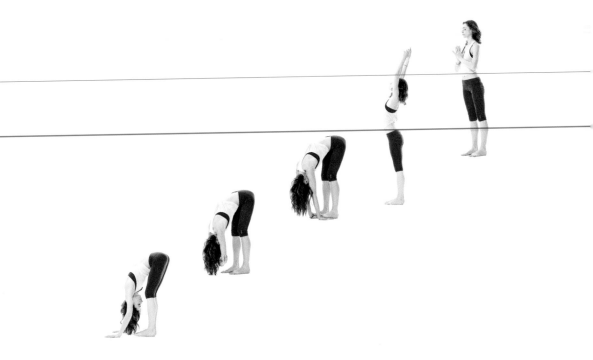

Walk your feet up to standing forward bend. Grab your elbows and relax your torso over your legs. Sway a bit side to side. Release your arms and step on your hands so the tops of your hands are on the ground, fingers pointing toward your heels. Soften your knees to take any pressure off your hamstrings. Relax your head and neck and hang here for several long, deep breaths. Release your hands and roll up to stand one notch at a time. When you make it up, take a big inhale and float your arms out and up. Press your palms together and bring your thumbs to your heartbeat. Soften here for a moment. Soften your knees. Relax your head and neck. Allow yourself to shift and drift from side to side or forward and back if that feels nice. Take a big inhale and lift your arms up overhead. Exhale and soften over your legs. Press your palms into the ground for support, bend your knees, and come into a squat. Lean toward your right and open your left arm upward, opening the front of your body. Roll around here if you'd like. When you're ready, go for the other side. When you're ready, bring your hands behind you on the ground for support and come to sit comfortably. Relax your hands on your thighs, close your eyes, and draw your attention inward. Stay here for a few long, deep breaths.

When you're ready, lean to your right side, reaching your left arm overhead. Roll around a bit here if that feels nice. Bring yourself back to center and go for the other side. Come back to center and crawl yourself forward. Relax your head and neck and hang here for a few long, deep breaths. Bring yourself back upright. Press your hands behind you on the

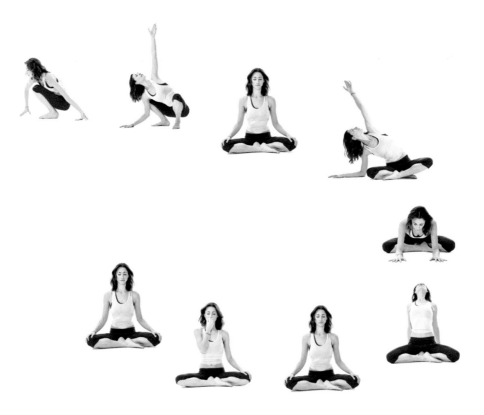

ground for support, take a big inhale, and lift your chest and hips up if that feels good. When you're ready, bring yourself back to seated.

   Come back to sit comfortably. We'll go for some **alternate nostril breathing** to calm the system. Make a peace sign with your right hand. Now curl those two fingers into your palm so you have your ring finger, your pinkie, and your thumb up. In between your ring finger and your thumb is just enough space for your nose. Close your left nostril by pressing with your ring finger. Close your eyes and take a big inhale through your right nostril. Close your right nostril with your thumb and hold the air for a moment. When you're ready, release your ring finger and let the air out your left nostril. Take a big inhale through your left nostril. Close the nostril with your ring finger and hold the air for a moment. Release your thumb and let the air out your right nostril. Repeat this for several minutes at your own pace. Relax your hands back on your thighs and come to easy breathing for a few moments. Stay with this for several long, deep breaths. If you notice your attention drifting, guide it right back to your breath. When you're ready, gently open your eyes.

I hope you feel as if you've let go of that stressful day and you're ready to enjoy a laid-back evening!

DISSOLVE STRESS

Sometimes the stress of life can feel a bit overwhelming. Constant deadlines, meetings, meet-ups, hangouts—life can be hectic. If you need more than a simple wind down, try this routine. It's set up to dissolve the mental and physical tension that has built up through your everyday life obligations and stresses. Easygoing, gentle movements will get your body moving, allowing the tension to roll right off, just like a refreshing waterfall running down your back. The fuller and deeper you breathe, the more space opens up. So breathe deeply and enjoy!

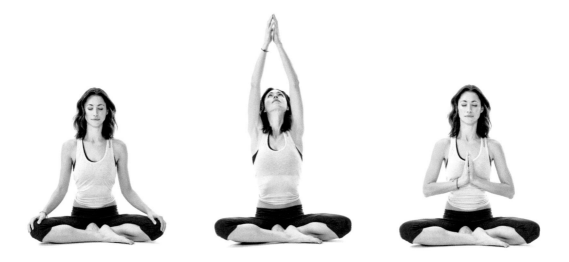

Start sitting, however you are comfortable. Close your eyes and rest your attention on your breath. If you notice your attention drifting, see if you can guide it right back to your breath. When you are ready, gently open your eyes.

Take a big inhale and lift your arms up overhead. Close your eyes, bring your palms together, and bring your thumbs to your heartbeat. Soften here for a moment. Take a big inhale through your nose. Long exhale out through your mouth. Twice more like that. Big inhale, long exhale. One more time. Big inhale, long exhale. When you are ready, gently relax your hands back on your thighs and open your eyes.

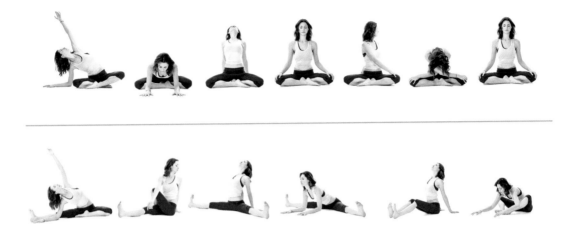

Staying soft, press your right hand on the ground beside you. Bend your torso to the side. Soften your elbow, resting your forearm on the ground. Stay here for a few moments. Bring your torso up through the center and do the same on the other side. Crawl your torso forward over your legs and relax here for a few long, deep breaths. Bring yourself back upright. Press your hands behind you on the ground and lift your chest up. Lift your hips up off the ground if that feels nice. When you're ready, bring yourself back, sit, and relax your hands back on your thighs.

Take a big inhale and lift your right arm up. Bring your arm down and twist to the left, pressing your right hand on your left thigh and your left hand behind you on the ground. Take a big inhale and lift your torso up. Exhale and twist around a little farther. When you're ready, bring your left hand up and around and grab ahold of your right knee so your hands are holding opposite knees. Relax your torso forward and let your head and neck relax. Hang here for a few long, deep breaths. Bring yourself back up to center and relax your hands on your thighs. Go for the other side.

Open your right leg out to your side, keeping your left leg tucked in. Lean toward your right side, pressing your right hand down to the ground. Soften your elbow and lean your forearm on the ground. Open your left arm up and overhead. Roll your torso open and hang here for a few long, deep breaths. Bring yourself back up to center and twist toward your left side. Press your right hand on your left thigh and press your left hand on the ground behind you for support. Take a big inhale and lift your torso up. Exhale and twist a little farther around to your left. Bring yourself back to the center and go for the other side.

Open your legs out to your sides so you feel a nice opening and can still breathe easily. Bring your fingertips behind you on the ground for support. Take a big inhale and lean back. Exhale and crawl yourself forward. Hang here for several long, deep breaths. Bring yourself back upright. Bring your legs in front of you and soften your knees a bit. Press your hands behind you for support. Take a big inhale and lean back. Exhale and crawl yourself forward. Hang here for several long, deep breaths. When you're ready, gently roll yourself back upright.

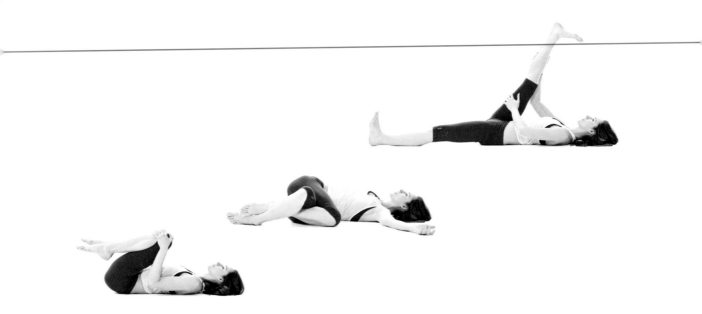

Soften your knees into your chest and roll down to your back. Cross your right leg over your left leg, and move your legs to your left side. Open your arms out to your sides and relax here in the twist for several long, deep breaths. Bring yourself back to center and go for the other side. Come back to center and unwind your legs. Hug your right shin into your chest and relax your left leg long on the ground. Open your right leg upward, holding your leg behind your thigh or knee if that feels good. Soften your knee to keep it easy on your hamstring. Hang here for a few long,

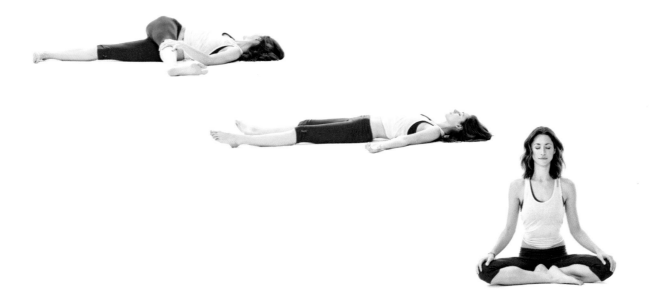

deep breaths. Relax your right leg across your body to your left and rest it toward the ground. Open your arms out to your sides and rest here for a few long, deep breaths. Come back to your center and go for the other side. Come back to center, stretch out a bit, and relax. Rest here for several long, deep breaths. Gently bring yourself up to sit. Close your eyes and rest your attention on your breath. Hang here for several long deep breaths. If you notice your attention drifting, guide it back to your breath. When you're ready, gently open your eyes.

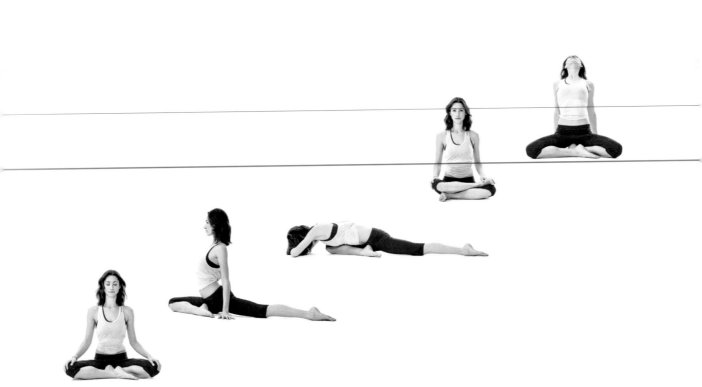

From sitting, lean into your right hip and bring your left leg behind you for pigeon. Hang here for a few long, deep breaths. Stay upright if that feels nice, or crawl yourself forward and rest for several long, deep breaths. Bring yourself back up to sitting, lean into your right hip, and bring your back leg around and stack your ankles and knees. If this doesn't feel good, rest your left leg in front of your right leg. Bring your hands behind you for support, take a big inhale, and lean back. As you exhale, crawl yourself forward and hang here for several long, deep breaths. When you're ready, bring yourself back to center and repeat on the other side.

Come back to sit comfortably. We'll go for some alternate nostril breathing to calm the system. Make a peace sign with your right hand. Now curl those two fingers into your palm so you have your ring finger, your pinkie, and your thumb up. In between your ring finger and your thumb is just enough space for your nose. Close your left nostril by pressing with your ring finger. Close your eyes and take a big inhale through your right nostril. Close your right nostril with your thumb and hold the air for a moment. Release your ring finger and let the air out your left nostril. Take a big inhale through your left nostril. Close the nostril with your ring finger and hold the air

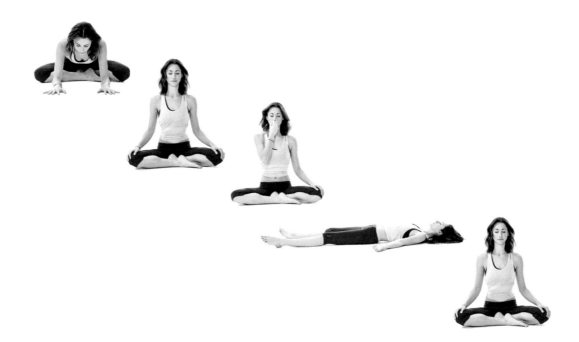

for a moment. Release your thumb and let the air out your right nostril. Repeat this for several minutes at your own pace. Relax your hands back on your thighs and come to easy breathing for a few moments.

With your eyes still closed, lie down and relax for several minutes. Gently bring yourself back up to sit. Draw your attention back to your breath. When you're ready, open your eyes.

Great job! I hope you feel de-stressed, fresh, and restored!

DETOX

We all have times in our lives when we feel extra stressed and our bodies and minds take the brunt of the battle for us. It could be from an unexpected life event or even from our own choices—we all make some fun mistakes, right? When your mind and body feel blah and you need a release, it's time to detox. This powerhouse healing routine is designed to unravel tension in the body and mind so you can return to feeling free and fantastic.

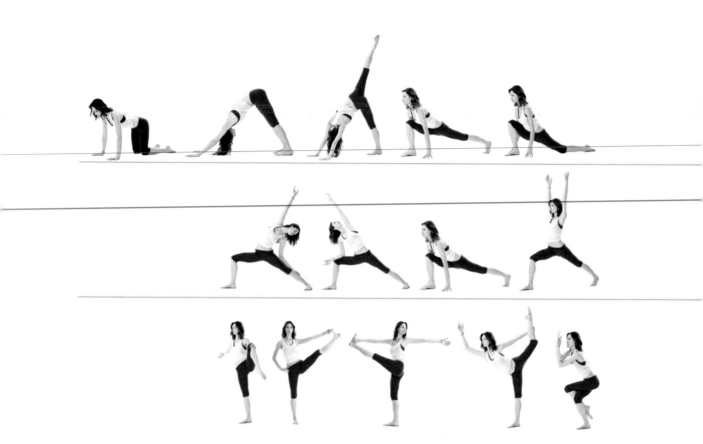

Come onto all fours. Spread your fingers wide, tuck your toes, and lift your hips up and back to down dog. Get comfortable here, moving around how it feels good to you. Take a big inhale and lift your right leg up and back to down dog split. Open your hips and belly if that feels nice. Exhale and step your foot through to low lunge. Ease your back knee to the ground and sway a bit here. Keeping your fingertips on the ground, shift your hips back to sit on your heel for runner's stretch. Relax your torso over your front leg and sway a bit here if you'd like.

Crawl yourself back to your low lunge, press your fingertips to the ground, take a big inhale, and lift your hips up as you relax your torso over your front leg. Hang here for a few long, deep breaths. Soften your knees, press your right fingertips to the ground, and open your left arm upward. Gaze upward if you'd like.

Press your left fingertips to the ground, take a big inhale, and lift your hips up and open your right arm and body toward your right side. Gaze upward if that feels nice for you. Bring your right fingertips down and hang your torso over your front leg for single leg forward bend. Hang here for a few long, deep breaths. Ground your back heel down, open your body toward your left, and lift your left arm up for triangle. Gaze upward if you want to. Soften your knees, reach your left arm back, press down through your legs, and lift up to stand, lifting your hips and arms up overhead. Exhale and soften to warrior 2. Take a big inhale and tip back to reverse warrior, sliding your left hand gently down your back leg and lifting your right arm up. Bring your body up and over to extended side angle, pressing your right forearm on your thigh and your left arm up and overhead. Roll your torso upward if that feels nice.

Come into low lunge. Sink your hips and sway a bit here. Press down through your legs, take a big inhale, and lift up to your high lunge. Press your palms together and

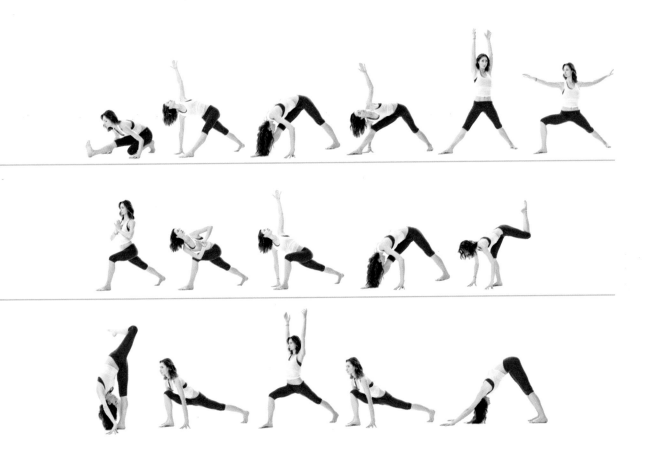

bring your thumbs to your heartbeat. Take a big inhale to lift up a bit. Exhale and twist toward your left, pressing your right elbow outside your left knee. Open your arms here, bringing your right fingertips to the ground inside your front foot, and open your left arm upward. Hang here for a few long, deep breaths. When you're ready, bring your fingertips to the ground on either side of your front foot and lift your hips up to single leg forward bend. Hang your torso over your legs for a few breaths.

Soften your knees, crawl your fingertips out in front of you, and lift your back leg up into warrior 3. Soften your knees and round up to stand, bringing your left shin in front of you for a squeeze. Grab ahold of your left big toe with the first two fingers of your left hand. Soften your knees to stay easy in the balance. If it feels good, extend your leg out in front of you. Extend your leg out to the side a bit if that feels okay. Bring your leg back to center. Grab ahold of your left knee or the outside of your ankle with your left hand. Take an easy twist to your left. Either hang here or open your leg out to the side, pressing your foot into your hand. Bring yourself back to center. Drop your left knee toward the ground and grab ahold of your ankle with your left hand. Gently press your calf into your hand for dancer. Hang here for a few breaths. When you're ready, bring your leg in front of you and wrap it around your standing leg for eagle. Wrap your left arm under your right arm as you sink through your hips and lift up through your fingertips. Unravel here and take a dive up and over your standing leg, bringing your fingertips to the ground for standing split. Relax your head and neck. Soften your knees and step your left leg back to low lunge. Take a big inhale and lift up to high lunge. Exhale back to low lunge and find your way back to down dog.

Repeat the movement phrase on the other side.

FLOW
OR GET STUCK

Watching water is so peaceful. As the waves come in and out, our tension drifts away. Simply by watching and allowing our minds to be involved in the easygoing flow of water, we soften, relax, and become peaceful. Let your movements be continuous like water. They can be slow and steady, or more rapid, but let them be fueled by your breath, not your muscles. When we move our bodies and hold ourselves tightly, we get stuck physically and mentally. Keep it easy and flow your way to the relaxing wave of nature that rests inside.

❀

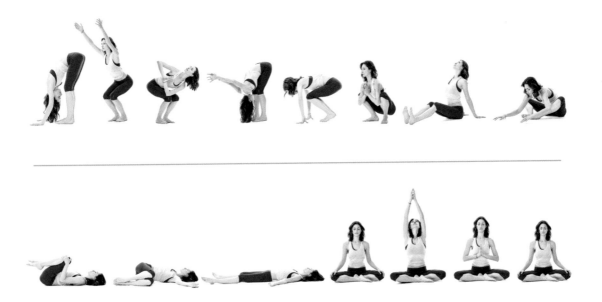

Take an easy walk up to the top of your mat and come into a standing forward bend. Relax your head and neck. Soften your knees, sink your hips, and come into chair, lifting your arms up. Exhale and twist toward your right side, bringing your left elbow outside your right knee. Take a big inhale back to chair. Exhale and twist toward your other side. Take a big inhale and come back to chair. Exhale and relax your torso over your legs. Interlace your hands behind you for a shoulder release. Release your hands, press your palms on the ground in front of you, and come into squat. Hang here for a few deep breaths to open. Bring your hands behind you on the ground and come to sit easy. Open your legs in front of you and soften your knees. Keeping your hands on the ground behind you, take a big inhale and open up your torso. Exhale and relax your torso over your legs. Hang here for a few long, deep breaths. Round yourself down to lie on your back, taking your knees along with you for the ride. Open your arms out to your sides and relax your knees over toward your right side. Hang here for several long, deep breaths and repeat on your other side. When you're ready, come back to center, stretch your legs out, and relax. Rest here for several long, deep breaths.

Gently bring yourself up to sit. Relax your hands on your thighs, close your eyes, and draw your attention inward. Take a big inhale and float your arms up and overhead. Press your palms together and bring your thumbs to your heartbeat. Soften here for a moment. Take a big inhale through your nose. Long exhale through your mouth. Twice more like that. Big inhale, long exhale. One more time, big inhale, long exhale. When you are ready, relax your hands on your thighs and gently open your eyes.

I hope you feel refreshed, released, and ready for a fresh start! I'm excited for you!

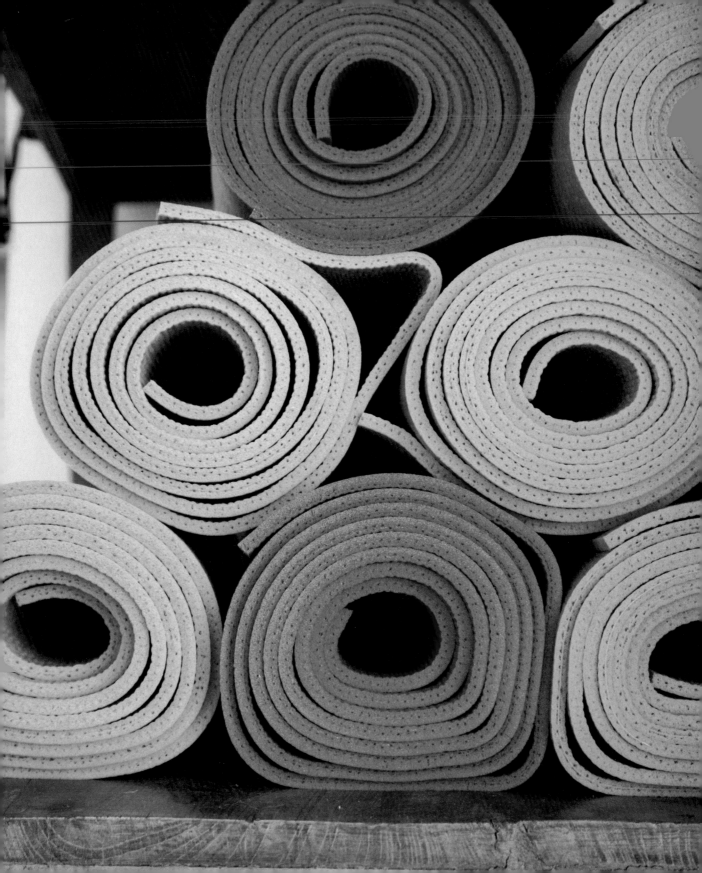

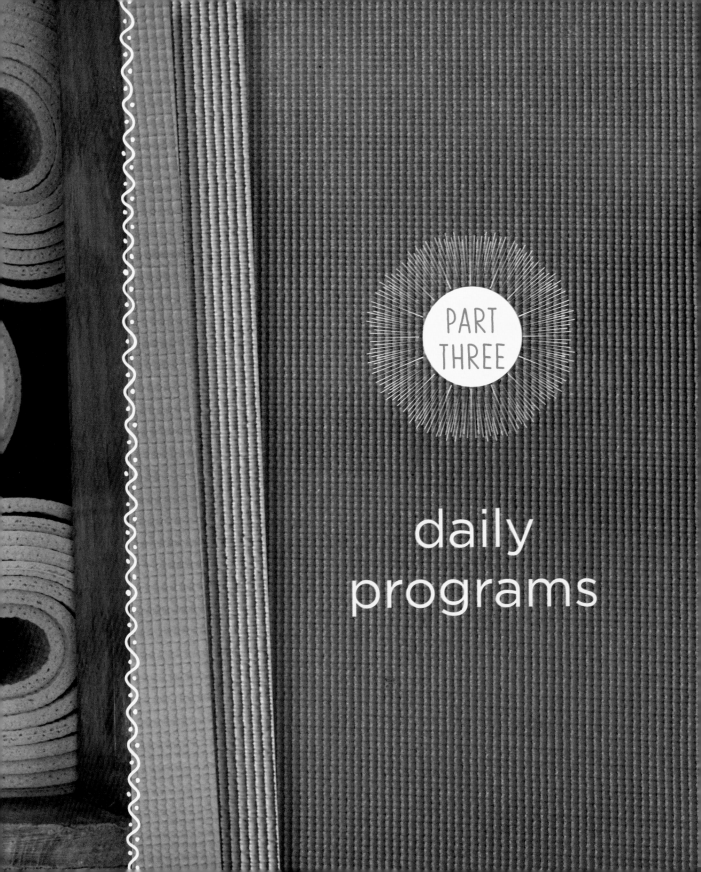

PART
THREE

daily
programs

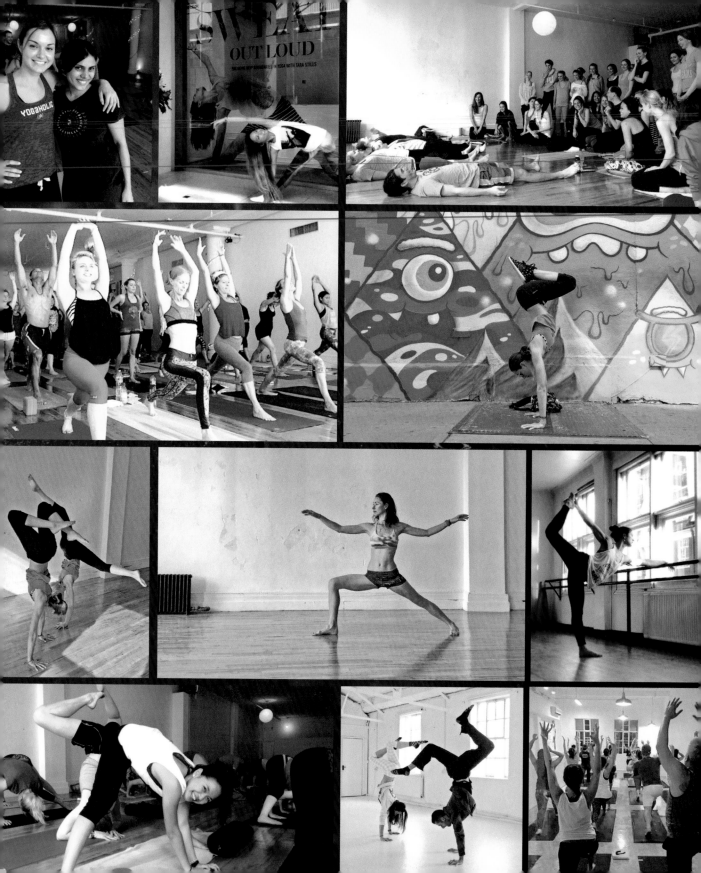

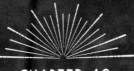

CHAPTER 12

YOUR 7-DAY JUMP START TO EASE

ALL this moving and living with ease, accomplishing more with less effort, and all the while leaving loads of room for creativity and feeling great sounds pretty awesome, right? It's one thing to observe and understand the process; it's another to do it—and to experience really nice, lasting, positive change. Luckily I've got you covered with a program that will incorporate Strala into your life—and you can start today! I laid out this plan for you with careful attention to help you ease into ease, while also giving you a good amount of challenge to keep things interesting. And it helps you wind things down properly so you feel rested and ready to take on each exciting day ahead.

The 7-day program consists of one full practice per day partnered with one or two shorter target practices and some moments of chill and check-in time. One of the great things about the practice of moving with ease is that you don't need a rest day! That said, if you feel like chilling out and need a break, feel free to modify the level of activity to best suit you.

To really get the most out of this program, I have three bits of advice:

1. **WRITE IT DOWN:** It is incredibly useful to write down how you feel each day before, during, and after the routines. Of course, the practices are physical, but there are mental and emotional components of moving with ease, and all that sensitizing is bound to open up and shift some things around. You might feel a burst of energy at different times of the day. You might feel more creative, connected, and in touch. You might experience a spontaneous rise in confidence grounded in good ideas and kindness. The possibilities are limitless.

2. **NOTICE OTHER HABITS:** Take notice of your non-working-out habits during the week. Hopefully the routines will set you in a superpositive, sustainable cycle of ridiculously awesome self-care. The habit of moving how it feels great for you is not-so-secretly designed to connect you to yourself. When you really see yourself, you'll make healthier choices in your day—because you'll notice their effects. I suspect you'll notice positive changes when it comes to preparing food and eating well, prioritizing rest, focusing your mind, letting stress roll off during the workday, and fostering healthy relationships. The results are, of course, different for each person, but you'll see some changes.

3. **SET A FEELING-BASED GOAL:** A lot of people set goals such as "I want to work out every day" or "I want to lose five pounds," but I find that these goals put undue pressure on you and often lead to frustration. So if you want to set a goal for yourself, set one like "I want to feel better and have less stress and more energy." Feeling-based goals are where it's at. When you choose your goal to feel great, taking the pressure off those frustration-inducing goals, amazing things happen. Often you reach or blow past those goals without even realizing it—just like in the practice when we focus on the process rather than the pose.

Okay! I think that's all you really need to know before jumping in. I'm excited for you! You're in for a fun ride! Breathe deeply and enjoy!

7-Day Jump Start

Here is your super boost starter week to moving how it feels great to move, sensitizing to all things awesome, and straight up radiating light. Tell your friends, family, co-workers, and local barista to get their shades out, because you are about to bust out some major light beams and positive vibes.

DAY 1

To gain ease of body, mind, and life, we begin, practice, and stay on the path of ease. We can't get to a place of ease from push, force, and struggle. This practice is designed to dissolve tension, create space, and sensitize you to feeling great so you extend that great feeling and choices into your life. Sounds great, right? Let's begin with a breath. We will always come back to the breath for fuel, energy, relaxation, and connection. Take a big, long, deep inhale. Let your exhale be longer, fuller, and deeper. Repeat this several more times, and take notice of how you feel. By simply bringing your attention to your breath, you become more calm, focused, and energized. By taking it a step further and lengthening and deepening the inhales and letting the exhales be even longer, you start the process of relaxation, ease, and creating space in your body, mind, and life. Take a big, deep breath and prepare to be in a luxurious process of ease.

MORNING

The first thing I'll ask you to do this morning is to really look inward. Reflect on how you've been feeling. The changes you'd like to see (remember to keep them based in feelings). Think about any topic that can remind you of how you feel in your life right now—your habits, your interactions with others, your outlook on life in general, your mood, your stress levels. If you want to write down what comes to mind, go for it. I'm going to ask you to reflect on your life again on Day 7, so be prepared—either with a solid memory or a nice written account. Now . . . prepare to get moving, feel better, and enjoy.

Take a moment to connect to your breath. Sit upright in bed, get comfy, and draw your attention inward. Spend a few moments breathing deeply.

Watch your inhales and your exhales as they come and go. If you notice your attention drifting, guide it right back to your breath. This simple practice is designed to set you up for the rest of the day. Whenever you feel stress pressing down on you, or space closing in, take a moment and draw your attention to your breath. You can do this while you're walking, at your desk, at home, or in the shower. When you need a moment, take a moment, and use it wisely. Come back to the breath. The fuller and deeper you breathe, the more room opens up. Space inside is limitless. Creating space inside will improve how you feel while you go about your day. Now get out there and enjoy!

AFTERNOON

Relax. Let's ease into Day 1 with a full routine that is simple enough to get your body moving and calm enough to release any tension. Roll out your mat and enjoy practicing Relax (page 181). If your day is too jammed and an afternoon practice isn't good timing for you, try fitting in Relax in the morning or evening to get connected and feeling great.

EVENING

As part two of your day begins, it's time to start the body and mind chill-out to get you into restore mode. Go for the simple practice of Wind Down (page 252) to transition your day to night.

BEDTIME

Congratulations on your first day! Did you notice any changes in your thoughts or your habits? Did your energy feel different? Maybe, maybe not, but good work on starting on a path to change. Now slide into the sheets and give yourself a few moments of deep breathing, right from bed. Sit up and get cozy and connect right to your breath. Hang here for several long, deep breaths, and then sleep well!

DAY 2

MORNING

Rise and shine! How are you feeling? I hope Day 1 was a success and you feel refreshed and ready for your day! Whether you are feeling energized straight out of the gate, or need a boost to get things cooking for you, try out Energize (page 151) and enjoy the day!

AFTERNOON

Whether you are feeling stress or not so much, taking some time to dissolve tension in the body and mind is a useful practice. Try out Dissolve Stress (page 256) and enjoy coming back to a refreshed you!

EVENING

Go for a few minutes of alternate nostril breathing (page 255) to dissolve stress and tension in the body, and bring you back to a calm, spacious state.

BEDTIME

Hop in those covers and move through the Better Sleep routine (page 250) and dream some great dreams!

DAY 3

MORNING

Good morning! How are you feeling? Is your body feeling good from the practices so far? Take note of how you feel. Try for the simple Wake Up routine (page 248) right from bed to get your morning moving right.

AFTERNOON

For a nice afternoon boost, try the Core routine (page 223) to really get into the middle of you and have a nice jolt of energy for the rest of the day.

EVENING

This evening, let's Dissolve Stress (page 256) again. This is always a good thing to do to keep you happy and in the flow. If you feel super-energetic, take it up a notch and do Basics (page 203). But remember—look inside and see what your body really needs. Either way, enjoy your evening!

BEDTIME

Sweet dreaming again! Try for some simple back to basics: do some easy meditation right from bed to cap off the night. Just focus on your breath.

DAY 4

MORNING

Hopefully you are really feeling the groove that all the physicality this week is bringing to you. Reconnect with the breath and do a few minutes of simple meditation right from bed to connect you back to all the good stuff inside.

AFTERNOON

For a simple afternoon break, try out the Detox routine (page 261) to hit the reset button.

EVENING

Let's keep the good vibes going and go for a simple practice of Wind Down (page 252).

BEDTIME

You've earned these sweet dreams tonight. Jump on in the sheets and go for the Better Sleep practice (page 250).

DAY 5

MORNING

Hope you are feeling fresh! Let's keep the morning easy and go for your Wake Up routine (page 248) right from bed.

AFTERNOON

If you can sneak away this afternoon, let's get in your Core routine (page 223) again, because I know you love that one so much.

EVENING

To wind down this day properly, let's do the full Relax practice (page 181) to give you some quality time with your breath-body connection.

BEDTIME

Hop on in that cozy bed and go for some simple meditation tonight—just breathe.

DAY 6

MORNING

Are you feeling it yet? Have you got any sudden lightbulb moments happening? Take some time to think about what you've been experiencing. Tap into how you're feeling, and then go for the Wake Up practice (page 248) right in bed. Enjoy the morning!

AFTERNOON

To keep the stress levels in check, move through the Dissolve Stress routine (page 256) wherever you are this afternoon.

EVENING

Let's kick it up a notch tonight and get in a solid Energize practice (page 151), because I know you are that strong.

BEDTIME

Let's wind it all down with your classic Better Sleep routine (page 250).

DAY 7

MORNING

Full sunshine is like bursting out of your head by now! Am I right? To close out your first week of practice, we're going to take it easy—simple, relaxing, fully enjoyable practices all day today. Let's start with Wake Up (page 248), right from the comfort of your own bed.

AFTERNOON

If you can, sneak in some quality time with your breath, because it feels so nice to reconnect.

EVENING

You've earned a solid Relax practice (page 181). Enjoy soaking up that luxurious deep breath of yours.

BEDTIME

Okay! Do you remember how I made you reflect on your life on Day 1? It's time to do it again. Tap into how you're feeling. Think about your experience. Did you notice any changes in your habits? Your energy? Your outlook? Your interactions with people? I hope you can see some amazing, positive changes. I know that I did when I started this process.

Now the topper of your jump start has arrived! Cap off your week with your Better Sleep routine (page 250). And then pat yourself on the back and settle in for a sweet night's sleep.

NOW WHAT?

Keep it going, of course! I'm sure you've learned quite a bit about how you feel with certain types of practices during each time of day. Keep your practice going in a way that is exciting and works for you. If you love to practice first thing in the morning, go for it. If you are more of a nighttime energy person, get your flow on at night. Try out different routines at different times of the day based on how you feel. By doing this, you'll find a nice program feels like a great addition to your awesome life. And if you're not quite ready to go out on your own, turn the page—my 30-day program is right there. I'm excited for you. Let me know how it goes!

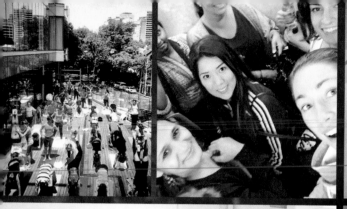
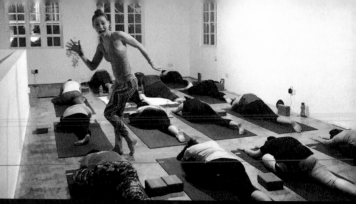
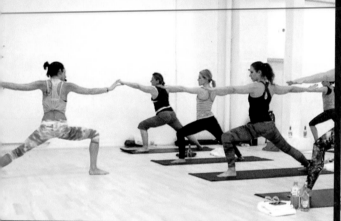
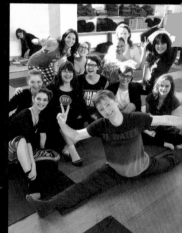
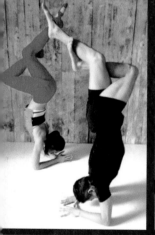
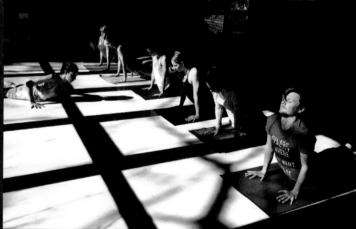
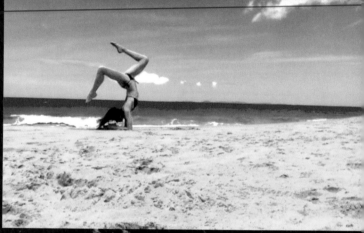
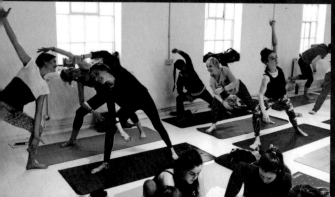
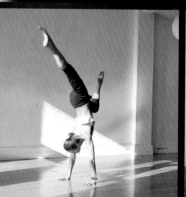
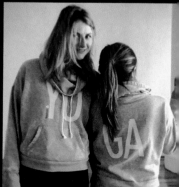

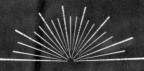

CHAPTER 13

YOUR 30-DAY GUIDE TO EASE

I have the privilege to see some of the same people come to classes at Strala day after day. And it's incredible to see and experience the lasting transformations they are making in their lives. Some started to practice because they wanted to feel better or reduce stress or simply get their bodies moving. Most of these folks have not only accomplished their initial goals but also gained so much more. And all of their changes have come from taking part in a consistent practice. With practice, unexpected shifts—big and small—happen sponta-neously. They start slowly, and then—wow! Life changes dramatically. But you have to show up day after day and make the goal to feel good. If you do, a posi-tive change will happen. Trust me. And usually it's something big, exciting, and life-changing. Whether you want to improve your mood, gain strength, allevi-ate pain, or amp up your health—or do all of the above—the transformation you experience may be more exciting than you can imagine. Focusing on the pro-cess instead of the outcome leaves room to reach and move past goals, blazing new and exciting territory along the way.

Because creating a consistent practice is such an important part of chang-ing your life, I've laid out this 30-day program. I know 30 days can feel like a big commitment, but I've tried to structure things in such a way that you can incorporate this program into your life without changing everything you do. Yeah, you'll likely need to get up a bit earlier—and instead of coming home and flopping down on the couch, I'll ask you to move your body. Just as in the 7-day jump start, I've outlined routines to do in the morning, afternoon, evening, and at bedtime. But I get that you're busy, so if you can't pull yourself away in the middle of the afternoon to do some yoga, feel free to simply sit at your desk and concentrate on your breathing for a bit. Or do some desk yoga—seriously, just Google it. The purpose of doing something for 30 days is to get yourself into a routine. Just remember—it's all about ease, so don't stress. If you miss a morn-ing because you woke up late or an afternoon because you were in a meeting, no big whoop. But if you want to see some amazing shifts in your life, do yourself a huge favor and give yourself 30 days with this practice. Something exciting will happen. There's no limit to what you can achieve—and you can do it with less effort than you might imagine.

Before you get started, you need to create space—both emotional and physical—to allow for things to shift. Like redecorating a home, we need to make room to make the awesome changes possible. Luckily you don't need to put your life on hold for the next 30 days to implement this program; how-ever, you may need to shift things around to make it a priority. Our lives are packed with events and responsibilities that we can't step away from. I get that. Stressed-out people come into the Strala studio in New York City every day, and they leave feeling better—and over time, they are better able to deal with the stress and frustration that are part of life. These people are wonderful examples of what can happen when we simultaneously practice self-care and keep up with the stuff of our lives.

My intention with this program for you is to find a sustainable balance between showing up for your practice and participating in your life. The practice is, after all, a tool to change your life. So it's best to have both experiences at the same time. Let them live next to each other. Let them play, intersect, and influence each other. How you are in your body and mind is how you live your life.

Reflecting on your experiences can be a powerful tool in this practice. Whether we share through writing or chatting, it's in our nature to connect and express ourselves. After a class at Strala, people usually hang around to talk with one another. It's not that it's a nightclub or a mixer; it's simply that people are simply feeling something and they're surrounded by other people feeling something, so they end up connecting. It's how we are made. When we have something to share, we share. It's natural. So as you're working your way through this program, write down your thoughts, creative ideas, and feelings, or talk about them with friends and family, if that's an option. Any form of sharing is a great tool to help process what's happening, which is why I recommend that you get a journal and do the writing exercises I've included in the program.

As you work your way through the program, you might notice that your habits start to change—for the better. This is because taking good care of yourself has a way of leading to taking even better care of yourself. A desire to eat healthier, work smarter, and live more brilliantly are all amazing effects of you spending this time on your mat and sensitizing yourself to how you feel.

One thing I'd like to emphasize before you start is that I want you to take it easy on yourself as you move through these next 30 days. There is no rush or hurry to get anywhere or achieve anything. The goal is simply to feel good. So if something in this program feels too intense for you, figure out something else to do. But don't be afraid to give something that seems intimidating a shot. Just remember to move with ease. You'll gain strength and the ability to achieve more by getting really comfortable moving.

All right! I think you're ready! Greatness is about to happen. You're about to go along for a ride designed to connect you right back inward. This ride will crack open your ability to sensitize yourself to how you feel, and program your system to deeply desire regular self-care. The possibilities are limitless! Let's do this!

DAY 1

MORNING

Let's get started by giving yourself a few extra moments to connect with your breath, right from bed. Sit up easy, close your eyes, draw your attention inward, and focus on your breath. When you notice your attention starting to shift or drift, guide your attention back to your breath. Stay with this for a few moments. Take a few moments to write a bit about your life as it stands now. How does your body feel? How are your energy levels? What foods do you eat? What foods do you want to lessen in your diet? What other shifts would you like to see?

AFTERNOON

Give yourself a break from whatever your day is bringing you, and go for the Dissolve Stress routine (page 256) to enjoy a nice boost of fresh energy for the rest of your day.

EVENING

Let's chill out this evening by going for the Wind Down routine (page 252). We're easing into the plan here and taking it slow to allow space for you to create new healthy habits in your routine.

BEDTIME

Take a few moments to connect with your breath right from bed. Sit up easy, close your eyes, draw your attention inward, and focus on your breath. When you notice your attention starting to shift or drift, guide your attention back to your breath.

DAY 2

MORNING

I hope you are feeling refreshed and energized. Let's keep it going with an Energize practice (page 151). Keep it easy and enjoy!

AFTERNOON

Take it easy this afternoon and find a bit of time to do some alternate nostril breathing (page 255) to shift your attention back inward and relax your body and mind for the rest of your day.

EVENING

It's time to Detox (page 261) to shed mental and physical tension.

BEDTIME

Keep it simple and take a few moments before bedtime to connect with your breath. It's a nice practice in the tub, shower, or even as you brush your teeth.

DAY 3

MORNING

Rise and shine! Let's get this morning moving easy in bed with your Wake Up routine (page 248).

AFTERNOON

Take a moment out of your day to connect with your breath. Go for a few minutes of alternate nostril breathing (page 255) to shift your attention inward, regain focus, and pump in some good energy!

EVENING

Get connected to the simple things of life and go for the Basics routine (page 203) this evening to unwind from the day and get you ready for rest.

BEDTIME

Hop in the sheets and go for the Better Sleep routine (page 250). Sweet dreams!

DAY 4

MORNING

Good morning! Get right into the groove with your Wake Up routine (page 248) right from bed.

AFTERNOON

To get a burst of strength and energy, go for the Core routine (page 223) this afternoon whenever your schedule allows.

EVENING

To wind down your day, go for the Dissolve Stress routine (page 256) to transition into night.

BEDTIME

Get in your pj's and go for some simple deep breathing, right from bed, to send you off to dreamland.

DAY 5

MORNING

Good morning to you! Let's switch it up a bit and hop on out of bed. Go for the Energize routine (page 151) to get your blood pumping!

AFTERNOON

Take a few moments break wherever you are and connect with your breath. Notice how the connection shifts the rest of your day.

EVENING

Let's wind down the day with Dissolve Stress (page 256). Ease into your evening and enjoy!

BEDTIME

Snuggle up in bed and go for a few minutes of alternate nostril breathing (page 255). Sweet dreams!

DAY 6

MORNING

Hope you are feeling fresh and ready for the day. Let's start with the Wake Up routine (page 248) right from bed.

AFTERNOON

Take some time for the Detox routine (page 261) to break up the day.

EVENING

As you're winding down for the night, go for Relax (page 181) to get a nice practice in to wrap up your day.

BEDTIME

Hope you are ready for a good night's sleep. Hop in bed and connect with your breath for a few moments.

DAY 7

MORNING

Good morning! Start the day off right with some simple meditation, right from bed.

AFTERNOON

Run through a Basics routine (page 203) to get your body moving.

EVENING

Wind down the day with Dissolve Stress (page 256). Enjoy the spaciousness in your body and mind.

BEDTIME

Hop up in bed and go for some alternate nostril breathing (page 255) to get you ready for sweet dreams.

DAY 8

MORNING

It's been one week! Congrats! I hope you're feeling amazing. And there's a way to find out: go back to your journal and read about how you felt when the program started. Do you feel different? Write about the changes you're noticing. And then get your morning moving with the Energize routine (page 151).

AFTERNOON

Take a moment to connect with your breath wherever you are. If you can squeeze in some alternate nostril breathing (page 255), that's even better.

EVENING

Let's wind down tonight with the Gentle routine (page 237).

BEDTIME

Snuggle up and get cozy with your breath for a moment. Go for your Better Sleep routine (page 250) right from bed.

DAY 9

MORNING

It's another beautiful day! Let's go for a few moments of simple meditation, right from bed.

AFTERNOON

Get moving from the middle to build some energy for the rest of the day. Go for the Core routine (page 223) and enjoy!

EVENING

Wind down any tension from the day with Dissolve Stress (page 256). Enjoy your evening.

BEDTIME

Hop up in bed and spend a few moments connecting with your breath. Then do a few moments of alternate nostril breathing (page 255) to calm you fully for a good night's rest!

DAY 10

MORNING

Rise and shine! Let's get this morning moving with your Energize routine (page 151). Keep it easy as you move and enjoy!

AFTERNOON

Go for a simple Detox routine (page 261) to wash off physical and mental tension from your day.

EVENING

Wind down the day by spending a few moments connecting with your breath.

BEDTIME

Hop up in bed and go for your Better Sleep routine (page 250). Sweet dreams!

DAY 11

MORNING

Good morning! Let's get moving with Wake Up (page 248) right from bed.

AFTERNOON

Roll off any tension from the day with the Dissolve Stress routine (page 256).

EVENING

It's always nice to check back in with your fundamentals. Let's go for the Basics routine (page 203). Remember to breathe deeply and fully.

BEDTIME

Get ready for great dreams by taking a moment to sit up easy in bed and connect with your breath for a few long, deep ones.

DAY 12

MORNING

Rise and shine! Let's hit the mat first thing today and roll out your Core routine (page 223). Enjoy the strength and focus you are building.

AFTERNOON

Sneak away a few moments for yourself to do some alternate nostril breathing (page 255) to ease the day.

EVENING

Keep the healing going with the Detox routine (page 261). Stay easy and enjoy.

BEDTIME

Take a few moments for your Better Sleep routine (page 250) before you head off to dreamland.

DAY 13

MORNING

You're still going strong! I hope you're feeling really great after all these days of new habits! Let's keep the energy going with your Wake Up routine (page 248) in bed.

AFTERNOON

Sometimes a nice, longer flow is a great break to the day. Go for Relax (page 181) to set the tone for the rest of your day.

EVENING

Take a few moments for alternate nostril breathing (page 255) to ease any tension that may have collected during your day.

BEDTIME

Go for your Better Sleep routine (page 250) to top off your day.

DAY 14

MORNING

Good morning! Let's start the day with some good vibes and your Energize routine (page 151).

AFTERNOON

Take a few moments to relax the tension by doing the Dissolve Stress routine (page 256).

EVENING

Try out the Detox routine (page 261) tonight to reset you back to the good stuff.

BEDTIME

Give yourself a few moments to unwind the day and connect with your breath. Sweet dreams.

DAY 15

MORNING

Wow! Are sparks flying out of your head yet? Congratulations! You're halfway through your 30-day program. I hope you are feeling great. Take some time to read through your notes about how you felt and then write some new ones. Once you're done celebrate with your Energize routine (page 151).

AFTERNOON

Take a few moments to simply connect with your breath. Enjoy the calm and focus.

EVENING

Let's go for your Wind Down routine (page 252) to let the day slide right off you.

BEDTIME

Cap this day off right with your now classic Better Sleep routine (page 250). You've probably added a few of your favorite moves into the mix by now!

DAY 16

MORNING

Rise and shine! Let's go for a few moments of deep breathing, right from bed, to start your day.

AFTERNOON

Schedule a date with yourself for a Core routine (page 223) today. Enjoy the strength you have and the strength you're building.

EVENING

Wind down any tension the day tossed at you with a nice Dissolve Stress routine (page 256). Breathe deep!

BEDTIME

Hop in the sheets and come right back to the breath. And then sleep like a baby.

DAY 17

MORNING

Are these practices a part of your life yet? I hope your energy levels are feeling great. Let's start today with some simple breathing to check in.

AFTERNOON

You've earned a nice Relax routine (page 181) to break up the day. Enjoy!

EVENING

Carve out some time for meditation tonight to connect and reflect on all you've been building these past couple of weeks!

BEDTIME

Get in your cozy bed and go for your Better Sleep routine (page 250). Dream well!

DAY 18

MORNING

Another awesome day ahead! Let's celebrate with a few moments of connecting with the breath.

AFTERNOON

Create some space for your Dissolve Stress routine (page 256) this afternoon.

EVENING

An evening Energize routine (page 151) is a nice way to mix up the day. Roll out your mat and enjoy!

BEDTIME

Take a few moments for alternate nostril breathing (page 255) right from bed to fully wind down the body and mind.

DAY 19

MORNING

Good morning! Let's hop right out of bed and go for your Core routine (page 223). You won't regret it!

AFTERNOON

Take a moment to connect with your breath and do some simple meditation.

EVENING

Let's restore a bit with your Gentle routine (page 237) this evening.

BEDTIME

Reset your system and prepare for great sleep with some alternate nostril breathing (page 255).

DAY 20

MORNING

You're in the home stretch and doing great! How are you feeling? Keep the energy going with Wake Up (page 248) right from bed.

AFTERNOON

Try on Detox (page 261) to shake off any stress from the day so far.

EVENING

Let's come back to your foundation, tap into body awareness, and celebrate how far you've come this month with your Basics routine (page 203).

BEDTIME

Take a moment to connect with your breath and let the day dissolve into the background. Sweet dreams!

DAY 21

MORNING

Welcome to another day of limitless possibilities! Start off by connecting with your breath, right from bed.

AFTERNOON

Take a breather and go for your Dissolve Stress routine (page 256) this afternoon.

EVENING

Let's go for Core (page 223) to keep the strength and body awareness building.

BEDTIME

Climb under the covers and do your Better Sleep routine (page 250). Enjoy.

DAY 22

MORNING

Good morning! Sit up in bed and connect with your breath for a few moments. Then grab that journal! It's the start of a new week. How are you feeling? Read through your old entries, write a new one, and then celebrate! Enjoy the day!

AFTERNOON

Slide out of the business of the day and give yourself time to Energize (page 151)! You'll never regret doing something positive and healthy for yourself!

EVENING

Relax, stay easy, and do your Dissolve Stress routine (page 256).

BEDTIME

Climb in your cozy bed and go for your Better Sleep routine (page 250) tonight. Feel free to add movements that feel great for you.

DAY 23

MORNING

Rise and shine! Let's start the day with some deep breathing right from bed.

AFTERNOON

Stay easy in your body and mind and go for your Dissolve Stress routine (page 256).

EVENING

Simmer down the evening with Wind Down (page 252).

BEDTIME

Go for Gentle (page 237) tonight and enjoy your sleep.

DAY 24

MORNING

Another gorgeous day! Let's get your morning moving with your Core routine (page 223).

AFTERNOON

Since you started out strong, let's keep it easy this afternoon. Enjoy your Relax routine (page 181).

EVENING

Get cozy for the night and spend some time connecting with your breath.

BEDTIME

Ahhhh . . . bedtime. Go for your Better Sleep routine (page 250), adding any of your newfound movements to help you wind down just right.

DAY 25

MORNING

You're in the home stretch of your program! I hope you are feeling more and more awesome each day. There really is no limit to how good you can feel! Feel free to shout "Yes!" if that is happening! It may be a little odd, but it celebrates your progress out loud. And that's awesome. Then keep the good vibes flowing with your Wake Up routine (page 248) right from bed.

AFTERNOON

Let's pump up the vibe today with a little afternoon Energize (page 151).

EVENING

Do some Detox (page 261) to dissolve any physical or mental blocks hanging around.

BEDTIME

Cap off this day with a few moments of deep breathing, right from bed.

DAY 26

MORNING

Rise and shine! Let's keep the strength up with Core (page 223) first thing!

AFTERNOON

Sneak in some time for your Gentle routine (page 237) and enjoy!

EVENING

Wind down today with a few moments of alternate nostril breathing (page 255).

BEDTIME

Hop in bed and do your Better Sleep routine (page 250). Sleep well!

DAY 27

MORNING

Goooood morning! We're almost there! Let's kick this day off with Energize (page 151) and start this day right.

AFTERNOON

Move into the afternoon with Detox (page 261) to drop extra mental and physical blocks that are standing in your way.

EVENING

Let's prepare for a peaceful evening with a few moments of connecting with the breath.

BEDTIME

Go for your classic Better Sleep routine (page 250) and have the best dreams yet!

DAY 28

MORNING

You're nearly done with this program—can you believe it? Hopefully you're well on your way to feeling great and setting some fantastic new habits for your life. Let's repeat what we did yesterday: Energize (page 151).

AFTERNOON

Take a moment for alternate nostril breathing (page 255) to enjoy connecting with your breath.

EVENING

Let's wind down a bit with Gentle (page 237).

BEDTIME

Hop up in your dream machine and spend a few moments connecting with your breath.

DAY 29

MORNING

Good morning! Let's start out with Basics (page 203) to set a great foundation for your day.

AFTERNOON

Set aside some time for your Detox routine (page 261).

EVENING

Take a few moments for your Wind Down routine (page 252) and enjoy the relaxation benefits!

BEDTIME

Bedtime is a great time after a long, enjoyable day. I hope you've had a great one so far. Let's top it off with Better Sleep (page 250).

DAY 30

MORNING

Your final day of this program has arrived! Let's start this day and celebrate with Energize (page 151)!

AFTERNOON

Keep the good vibes going by taking a few moments to connect with your breath in meditation.

EVENING

Roll any tension off you from the day with Dissolve Stress (page 256).

BEDTIME

You've done it! How do you feel? Has something happened, shifted, or grown from this now-regular habit of amazing self-care, moving with ease, and reflecting on how you feel? All this sensitizing is bound to lead somewhere incredible. Read through your journal. I'm sure you'll notice that oodles of things have changed. Take a few moments to be grateful for anything that has shifted. And then congratulate yourself. You're amazing! You deserve everything you've made happen. Once you're ready, jump in bed, do your Better Sleep routine (page 250), and drift off to sleep, content in the knowledge that you can do whatever you set your mind to.

I hope this program has helped you figure out just how to fit movement into your life—and how crazy awesome it can be. Its goal was to connect you back to you, so you could find all those special sparks that make you you and light them up like fireworks. Hopefully all this moving with ease and connecting to the breath roots you in to the best stuff of you and gives you the strength and courage to create your own program. With consistent practice, you can live an actualized life and tap into the infinite possibilities that are available to you.

Thank you for taking such great care of you. The more you take care of you, the more we all benefit. Stay easy and enjoy!

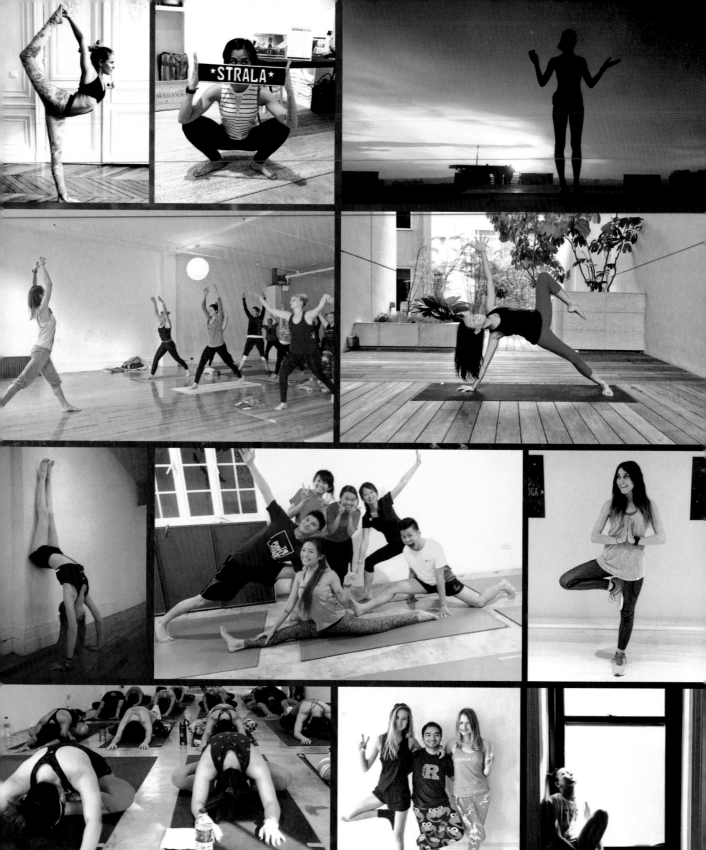

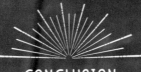

CONCLUSION

FINAL WISHES
FOR YOU

Every time I walk into the studio and connect with a group of people, I get excited. Helping people find freedom and ease on and off the mat connects me to my intuition and awareness, and helps me feel useful in the world. If I can help you feel better, you are able to do better in your life, and that's awesome. My goal is to help anyone who happens to cross my path. I want to help everyone dissolve tension, build awareness, and connect to a sense of purpose through moving intuitively with ease.

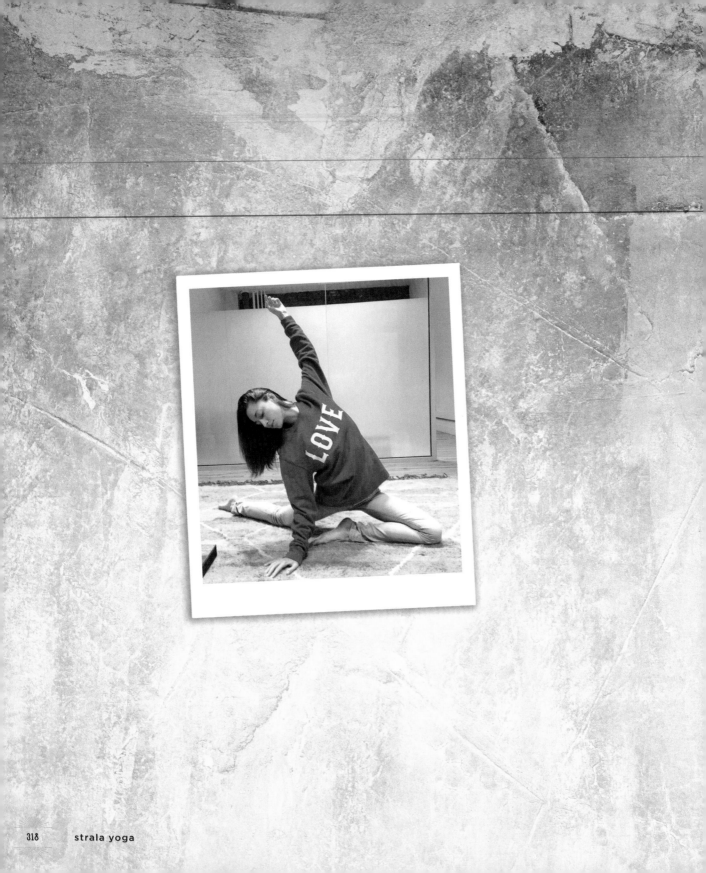

I've seen the practice of Strala work time after time in ways that are incredibly unique and almost unbelievable. The stories of transformation I have had the pleasure of hearing call for big hugs, massive celebrations, and often happy tears. It's not the poses, the movement, or the breathing that creates the magic; it's the process of moving through simple and challenging feats with ease, allowing space for your body to restore and your mind to clear, expand, and focus.

I feel so grateful to have found this practice. Having tools that help me connect to myself, follow my intuition, and live with ease is a precious gift. I'm excited about the possibilities we all have resting inside, waiting to be discovered. Strala is a practice of removing tension, unhealthy patterns, and movements that prevent us from living out our potential. When we focus on the process and move with ease naturally from where we are, our range of possibilities expands. And the results often come quicker and bigger than we can even imagine.

Once you connect to your awesome place and find your natural way, please take what you've learned and share it with those around you. Hopefully they will learn to feel better too. When you feel great, it's impossible not to want to help others. Share your lessons, your tips, your story, and your practice far and wide. Find ways to communicate and offer useful suggestions for those who ask. And for those who don't ask, know that by living with grace and ease, you're inspiring joy in everyone and lifting them up with your peaceful radiance. You are a shining example of how to live well. So keep the good vibes spreading! Together we can improve things a bit.

Come find me and tell me what happens! I can't wait to hear about your adventures.

❊ love, Tara ❊

ACKNOWLEDGMENTS

Laura Gray, thank you for really getting the Strala vibe and all its details that make the magic happen, and putting up with me project after project.

Forever thank you to Patty Gift, Reid Tracy, Sally Mason, Richelle Fredson, and the whole Hay House family, for giving me such a great and nurturing home, being awesome people to learn from, and for being real life friends.

Charles McStravick, these books look fabulous because of you. Thank you for your time, creativity, talent, and being super rad.

Sam Berlind, thank you for the leaning, support, and just the right balance between confidence and skepticism that keeps me improving.

To all the Strala Guides, studio owners, supporters, and people who believe that an easygoing approach is our best way to accomplish the greatest of challenges, this is about you. Thank you for the inspiration and guidance through your passion and tireless practice.

Jason and Colleen Wachob, through all the evolutions and revolutions, thank you for your friendship, guidance, and support.

Mike, well you know, it's a together thing.

ABOUT THE AUTHOR

Tara Stiles is the founder and owner of Strala, the movement system that ignites freedom. Thousands of guides are leading Strala classes around the globe in partner studios, gyms, and clubs. Tara partners with W Hotels on FIT with Tara Stiles, a global program bringing Strala Yoga classes and healthy recipes to W properties around the globe. She is a collaborator with Reebok, working closely with the design team on their Reebok Yoga lifestyle line, and has authored several best-selling books including *Slim Calm Sexy Yoga*, *Yoga Cures*, and the most recent, *Make Your Own Rules Cookbook*. Tara supports the Alliance for a Healthier Generation, President Clinton's initiative to combat childhood obesity, bringing Strala classes to more than 20,000 participating schools. Strala's flagship studio is in downtown New York City.

Visit: tarastiles.com.

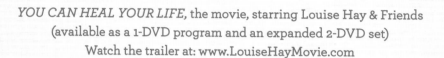

HAY HOUSE
TITLES
OF RELATED
INTEREST

YOU CAN HEAL YOUR LIFE, the movie, starring Louise Hay & Friends
(available as a 1-DVD program and an expanded 2-DVD set)
Watch the trailer at: www.LouiseHayMovie.com

THE SHIFT, the movie, starring Dr. Wayne W. Dyer
(available as a 1-DVD program and an expanded 2-DVD set)
Watch the trailer at: www.DyerMovie.com

LIGHT IS THE NEW BLACK:
A Guide to Answering Your Soul's Callings and Working Your Light,
by Rebecca Campbell

MIRACLES NOW:
108 Life-Changing Tools for Less Stress, More Flow, and Finding Your True Purpose,
by Gabrielle Bernstein

PERFECTLY IMPERFECT:
The Art and Soul of Yoga Practice,
by Baron Baptiste

RADICAL SELF-LOVE:
A Guide to Loving Yourself and Living Your Dreams,
by Gala Darling

All of the above are available at your local bookstore,
or may be ordered by contacting Hay House (see next page).

WE HOPE YOU ENJOYED THIS HAY HOUSE BOOK. IF YOU'D LIKE TO RECEIVE
OUR ONLINE CATALOG FEATURING ADDITIONAL INFORMATION ON HAY HOUSE BOOKS AND PRODUCTS,
OR IF YOU'D LIKE TO FIND OUT MORE ABOUT THE HAY FOUNDATION, PLEASE CONTACT:

Hay House, Inc., P.O. Box 5100, Carlsbad, CA 92018-5100
(760) 431-7695 or (800) 654-5126
(760) 431-6948 (fax) or (800) 650-5115 (fax)
www.hayhouse.com® • www.hayfoundation.org

Published and distributed in Australia by:
Hay House Australia Pty. Ltd., 18/36 Ralph St., Alexandria NSW 2015
Phone: 612-9669-4299 • Fax: 612-9669-4144 • www.hayhouse.com.au

Published and distributed in the United Kingdom by:
Hay House UK, Ltd., Astley House, 33 Notting Hill Gate, London W11 3JQ
Phone: 44-20-3675-2450 • *Fax:* 44-20-3675-2451 • www.hayhouse.co.uk

Published and distributed in the Republic of South Africa by:
Hay House SA (Pty.), Ltd., P.O. Box 990, Witkoppen 2068
info@hayhouse.co.za • www.hayhouse.co.za

Published in India by:
Hay House Publishers India, Muskaan Complex, Plot No. 3, B-2, Vasant Kunj,
New Delhi 110 070 • Phone: 91-11-4176-1620 • Fax: 91-11-4176-1630 • www.hayhouse.co.in

Distributed in Canada by:
Raincoast Books, 2440 Viking Way, Richmond, B.C. V6V 1N2
Phone: 1-800-663-5714 • Fax: 1-800-565-3770 • www.raincoast.com

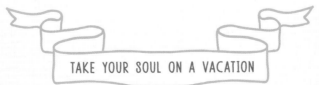

TAKE YOUR SOUL ON A VACATION

Visit www.HealYourLife.com® to regroup, recharge, and reconnect
with your own magnificence. Featuring blogs, mind-body-spirit news,
and life-changing wisdom from Louise Hay and friends.

Visit www.HealYourLife.com today!

FREE E-NEWSLETTERS FROM HAY HOUSE, THE ULTIMATE RESOURCE FOR INSPIRATION

Be the first to know about Hay House's dollar deals, free downloads, special offers, affirmation cards, giveaways, contests, and more!

 Get exclusive excerpts from our latest releases and videos from *Hay House Present Moments*.

 Enjoy uplifting personal stories, how-to articles, and healing advice, along with videos and empowering quotes, within *Heal Your Life*.

 Have an inspirational story to tell and a passion for writing? Sharpen your writing skills with insider tips from *Your Writing Life*.

Sign Up Now!

Get inspired, educate yourself, get a complimentary gift, and share the wisdom!

http://www.hayhouse.com/newsletters.php

Visit www.hayhouse.com to sign up today!

 HAY HOUSE

 HAYHOUSE RADIO *radio for your soul*

HealYourLife.com

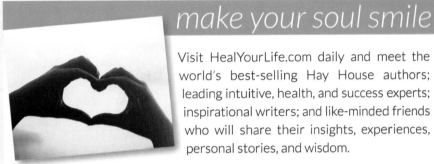

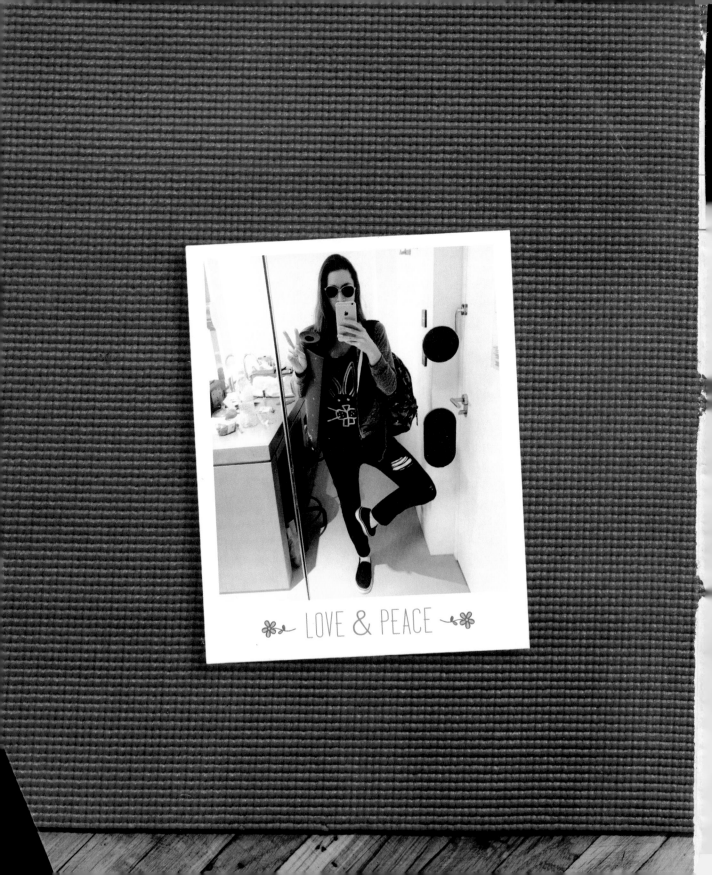